The Image of Madness

The Image of Madness

The Public Facing Mental Illness and Psychiatric Treatment

Editors

José Guimón, Geneva
Werner Fischer, Geneva
Norman Sartorius, Geneva

36 figures and 34 tables, 1999

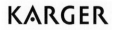

KARGER   Basel · Freiburg · Paris · London · New York ·
New Delhi · Bangkok · Singapore · Tokyo · Sydney

••••••••••••••••••••••••

José Guimón
Werner Fischer
Norman Sartorius

Department of Psychiatry (HUG)
2, chemin du Petit-Bel-Air
CH–1225 Chêne-Bourg/Geneva (Switzerland)

Library of Congress Cataloging-in-Publication Data
The image of madness / editors, José Guimón, Werner Fischer, Norman Sartorius.
Includes bibliographical references and index.
1. Mental illness – Public opinion. 2. Mental illness – Chemotherapy – Public opinion. I. Guimón, J.
II. Fischer, Werner. III. Sartorius, N.
[DNLM: 1. Mental Disorders – psychology. 2. Attitude to Health. 3. Public Opinion. WM 31 I31 1999]
RC455.2.P85I46 1999 362.2 – dc21
ISBN 3–8055–6846–0 (hardcover: alk. paper)

© Copyright 1999 by S. Karger AG, P.O. Box, CH–4009 Basel (Switzerland)
www.karger.com
Printed in Switzerland on acid-free paper by Reinhardt Druck, Basel
ISBN 3–8055–6846–0

Contents

Contents   VI

Introduction

Negative moral judgments seem to have been a constant fixture in the way societies and cultures have regarded groups displaying deviant behavior. This is particularly true of the mentally ill who, during the early nineteenth century, underwent classification into categories susceptible to psychiatric treatment. 'Medicalizing' this particular form of deviancy has not led to an alleviation, or even a neutralization, of the negative responses it inspires. On the contrary, stigmatization has spread to psychiatry itself which was made responsible for controlling and correcting its manifestations. This remains true today since the term 'psychiatrization', despite some semantic modifications, is unanimously defined as a derogatory description of behavior, attitude and thought.

Psychiatric deinstitutionalization, beginning in the 1950s, did not merely open a door onto the outside world and society; it multiplied the contacts between the mentally ill and persons considered to be normal. Stigmatization which had originally centered on an entity, a concept – madness – and on its almost exclusive domain – the psychiatric hospital, thus shifted, influencing public conduct towards the mentally ill in the community, relations with and attitudes towards them. This passage into open society conditioned other transformations, for example the creation of differentiated negative stereotypes resulting from specific behavior, specific psychopathology. But the most radical stigmatization systematically victimizes schizophrenics who seem to display the greatest number of traits which lead to rejection and social exclusion.

Studies on social representations and public attitudes towards mental illness, on stigmatization and the exclusionary process from which patients suffer, were carried out over this same period in both psychiatry and the social sciences. Two principal orientations emerged to structure perspectives: 'labeling' first theorized by Lemert and Scheff in the 1950s and 1960s and the interactionist theory primarily defended by Goffman and Mechanic. All of the studies, the most representative of which are quoted in this volume, report the general prejudice against the mentally ill whatever the context: different cultures, urban or rural regions, care facilities, target audiences or general public.

The present work evaluates the current status of social stereotypes associated with mental illness as well as examining attitudes towards psychiatry in general. It also investigates the changes that have occurred in this area. Our endeavor appears even more timely as the World Psychiatric Association has instigated a program which aims to lessen the stigmatization of the mentally ill and forestall their exclusion from many spheres of life. Finzen reminds us, first of all, of the pivotal role played by schizophrenia in popular stereotypes of mental illness and in the mechanisms of stigmatization. Endowed with occult powers, it is interpreted as a mysterious malediction, bizarre and inexplicable. The schizophrenic suffers from total and absolute vilification as if the whole of his or her being were infected, ravaged by illness.

The idea of the outgrowth of the illness is probably linked to the predominant public image of schizophrenia: a personality disintegrated, split into several disjointed elements, as Angermeyer and Matschinger show in their analysis of the social representations of schizophrenia. Pont also points out that the stigma adds to the burden of the primary disorder to create schizophrenia's secondary illness which violates not only the patient's identity, but distorts the image they have of themselves. The stigma then appropriates all the links to mental illness: discrediting patient associations, care facilities and psychiatric professionals.

The danger represented – or thought to be represented – by psychiatric patients is another fixture of the labeling process. According to various studies, perception of the danger represented by the mentally ill is inversely proportionate to familiarity: the more contact there is, the less mental patients are deemed threatening. Experience with mental illness, either directly or indirectly, also diminishes stereotypes about perceived danger. Brändli draws our attention to the fact that subjects and their entourage tend to confine the social interaction of someone who is mentally ill to the family circle, a restricted network of close friends and the family doctor, in order to avoid embarrassing situations. They appear to validate outright public fears of contact with the mentally ill, reconciling themselves to prejudice and thereby contributing to and reinforcing stereotypes.

It is interesting to note – as Goerg et al. show – that the logic behind reactions to the mentally ill themselves can be discovered in the description of social situations which represent less obviously visible forms of deviant behavior and which are not readily considered to be manifestations of illness.

Angermeyer and Matschinger reported that the general public does not a priori differentiate between the different psychiatric disorders (schizophrenia, depression and panic disorder) or between the various psychotropic medications prescribed for them. This is, however, not the case when the public is confronted by deviant situations in daily life. Preference is then given to psychiatric intervention, even recourse to psychotropic medication, more often to counter violence than for odd behavior or symptoms of withdrawal. Psychiatry therefore finds its legitimacy in situations that lend themselves most readily to stigmatization.

Yllá and Hidalgo find analogous results in the general public and among psychology students for their representation of the professions of psychiatry and psychology. Psychiatrists were assigned the treatment of the mentally ill and those patients having psychological problems associated with somatic illness. Psychologists were expected to resort exclusively to psychology to resolve difficulties for persons who were in otherwise good physical health. In a more general fashion, Sartorius supports the notion that the social stigmatization of mental patients is reinforced and reproduced in the health-care system. Several indices confirm this: lesser resources allocated to psychiatry than to somatic medicine, more restricted access to treatment, lower standards in psychiatric practice, absence of research which would permit the elaboration of strategies to prevent psychiatric disorders and their effects.

For the study on representations of mental illness, two types of methodology were principally used. In the first instance, the technique of using vignettes elaborated by Star was employed to create a portrait constructed out of the most salient diagnostic features of, for example, schizophrenia, anxiety disorder and affective disorders. The second method of research utilized attitude scales of which the principal and most commonly used is the OMI scale (Opinions about Mental Illness) of Cohen and Struening. This scale, many of whose variations have been formulated and adapted in the context of specific research, present a factorial structure which has shown itself to be stable in different studies.

From a methodological point of view, these two research trends have formed the object of a certain amount of criticism, according to which both the vignettes and the attitude scales confront interview subjects with scenarios based in clinical psychiatry and the institutional management of patients. Answers would therefore be prompted by certain characteristics whose pertinence resides in underlying psychopathology rather than in the logic applied to social interaction and the cultural significance of daily life. Other remarks stress the fact that, among subjects interviewed, few have ever encountered the situations presented in the questionnaire or mentioned in the scales; this could engender hypothetical reactions and attitudes which may diverge very strongly from real-life situations. Finally, these methods would give credency to the notion that mental illness is a singular concept that does not include differing mental states.

New research perspectives have been applied and are described in this volume. Hillert et al. consider that the image of mental illness conveyed by clinical vignettes is much too general and lacking in differentiation. They propose clearly distinguishing between cognitive and affective dimensions, thus building profiles which take into account the disparate identities of psychiatric patients. These profiles describe situations which correspond most closely to the distinctions subjects make about different disorders under varying social conditions. Schurmans and Duruz propose abandoning the approach which primarily attempts to assess how the lay public connects to scientific knowledge and mental health professionals. This reorientation should be directed towards examining the compatibility and antagonism that exists between lay knowledge and professional expertise. Therapeutic relationships furnish a prototype. These authors note that 'Therapists should appreciate that all knowledge is elaborated from pre-existing conceptions and knowledge that should be taken into consideration and therefore unveiled.' This is true not only of therapeutic relations, but also of any predicament where disparate theories and knowledge come into confrontation – whether the problem is mental illness itself or compliance, as thoroughly analyzed by Thorne.

Certain articles contained in this volume touch on the question of whether attitudes on, and representations of mental illness and patients have changed or if, on the contrary, we are witnessing the endurance of negative stereotypes. Eker and Öner champion recourse to experimental methods, especially to change attitudes towards the mentally ill. Wolff et al. describe the results of such an experimental study. They note that: 'The results of the follow-up survey suggest that although the public education intervention may have, at best, only a modest effect on knowledge, it is associated with an improvement in overall attitudes and behavior toward the mentally ill. ... However, the education campaign did not in itself lead directly to less fearful attitudes, whereas contact with patients did. It is likely, therefore, that the campaign exerted its effect on overall attitudes indirectly by encouraging contact with patients.' Yllá and González-Pinto observe practically no change in attitudes towards mental patients among medical students. No significant difference was noted between the two types of intervention: theoretical formative and experiential.

According to Eker and Öner, a major reason for the absence of modification in attitudes may reside in the fact that stereotypes and negative attitudes are assimilated at an early stage of socialization. They form part of the very basis of our culture. Thus, effectively, this is not simply a question of isolated prejudice. In the study of Fischer et al., it is shown that we are faced with belief systems encompassing not only illness and psychiatric patients, but also psychiatric therapy. Warner views the situation from the same angle. After having analyzed the fundamental aspects of alienation (meaninglessness, powerlessness, normlessness and estrangement from society and work), he shows how these problems may be dealt with to lessen their effects: humanizing and normalizing techniques which empower patients, alternatives to hospitalization, professional activity to promote feelings of worth and self-esteem, consumer-run programs.

Comments made about the general public image of mental illness also apply to opinions and attitudes about psychiatric treatment, particularly psychotropic medication. Angermeyer and Matschinger point to the important hiatus between popular beliefs and current scientific knowledge. Firstly, the public does not differentiate between neuroleptics and other psychotropic drugs (anxiolytics and antidepressants for example) and has very negative attitudes towards them. The notion is widely held that these drugs are addictive or lead to dependency and should only be used as a last resort.

Attitudes towards psychotropics and medication in general seem to be influenced by their own logic, independent of any beliefs about the origin of mental illness or its evolution. The analysis of different therapeutic possibilities reveals, in the study by Fischer et al., a new aspect: bias against and refusal of psychotropics constitute indications of a more general opposition to medicine itself and psychiatry in particular. Effectively, people who refuse psychotropics as a therapeutic option also tend to disregard both individual psychotherapy and family therapy, preferring natural means and relaxation techniques. In this area as well, studies have been carried out on modifications in attitude for health-care professionals such as, for example, that of Hillert et al. among medical students. An altered outlook seems a certainty as students advance through the syllabus. But the question of ascertaining which processes effect these changes should be further investigated.

In improved acceptance of psychotropic medication lies crucial patient compliance; from numerous studies we have learned that it is weak and problematic. The chasm dividing therapeutic conviction from patient behavior seems so wide that the usual recommendations (a relationship of trust, accessible language in communicating with the patient, involvement of the entourage) do not appear to rectify this therapeutic deficit. In contrast, Eguiluz et al. devised a psychoeducational program for groups of schizophrenic patients with the aim of promoting improved compliance in order to decrease risks of relapse. When compared to a control group, those patients in the program were significantly less frequently readmitted to hospital.

New research directions allow us to better understand this phenomenon. After having analyzed recourse to psychotropics in various countries and the factors significantly associated with their prescription, Guimón et al. place difficulties with compliance in the context of the patient's attitude towards his or her disorder. Thus, poor compliance may be a sign of denial of illness or an insufficient consciousness of it. The patient may stop taking medication to 'test' his or her mental state in the absence of psychopharmacological intervention. Alternatively, the therapist may unconsciously contribute to a patient's lack of compliance. Spagnoli also notes that the benefits of neuroleptics are often better perceived by therapists and a patient's entourage than by patients themselves. She proposes an interpretation of the significance of taking or refusing this medication. Effectively, medication confirms the illness and hints at its severity, constantly reminding a patient – even when he or she is feeling better – of its existence. Additionally, when responsibility for supervision of compliance falls to the entourage, it is symbolic of the denial of a patient's autonomy. Warnings about noncompliance affix themselves to other judgments of inadequacy, thereby corroborating not only psychiatric disorder but also reinforcing social stereotypes.

Draine extends the analysis of the problem of compliance to persons in the patient's entourage, studying their own therapeutic discipline. Therefore, compliance with medication should not be considered merely intrinsic to patients or to a psychiatric disorder. Attitudes towards prescription drugs would thus form part of a collective context which influences – as much as personal prejudice – the decisions patients take with regard to their medication.

Finally, DiMatteo proposes that the patient be implicated as much as possible in the decisions taken by the physician, that the patient be granted the right to be an active partner in issues of consent and informed choice. For these aspects, in analogy to the findings of Schurmans and Duruz on representations parents make of their child's psychiatric disorder, Thorne defines noncompliance not in the terms of a senseless act, but rather as a rational choice based on a patient's knowledge and experience. In this domain, patients also have an obvious expertise. Such questions can no longer be considered as a lack of submission on the patient's part to the physician's greater authority and knowledge; they have become bargaining chips between the therapist and patient in negotiating the different aspects of illness where the management of medication becomes an integral issue.

These changes in perspective concern patient compliance and its relationship to treatment and psychotropic drugs in particular. They are an element of the sea change which would narrow the breach, extensively documented in the literature, between mental illness and normality. Studies and strategies of action to counteract discrimination against the mentally ill have gained momentum, not only in medicine and psychiatry, but also in the sociopolitical arena and in the advocacy movement. The goal of these programs is to better educate the general public, increasing community involvement, knowledge and awarness of mental illness throughout the health-care and educational systems as well as changing the laws that sustain, or even reinforce the stigmatization and exclusion which effectively constitute the major obstacle to efforts to develop community medicine and mobilize resources in order to promote an inclusive society and better serve the needs of patients and their families.

José Guimón
Werner Fischer
Norman Sartorius

Guimón J, Fischer W, Sartorius N (eds): The Image of Madness. The Public Facing Mental Illness and Psychiatric Treatment. Basel, Karger, 1999, pp 1–12

....

Attitudes toward Mental Illness among the General Public and Professionals, Social Representations and Change

Doğan Eker, Bengi Öner

Department of Psychology, Middle East Technical University, Ankara, Turkey

The need for the treatment of mental disorders outside of hospitals and within their communities is well recognized today. This is especially the case in developing countries which typically have limited resources for health care. Even in a developed country like the USA it was reported by Beigel [1] that the resources for individuals with significant mental disorders were rapidly shrinking.

With the shift of emphasis from centralized hospitals to community-based care, the reactions of the community, including the family, friends, relatives, the neighborhood, and the mental health professionals at various levels, have gained in importance [2–4]. The community's, particularly the family members', perception of and attitudes toward mental illness and the mentally ill have a significance regarding the prevention, early detection and community treatment of mental illness. The family members' and other significant persons' definitions of and attitudes toward mental illness must be known for the successful introduction and utilization of community-based mental health care. In addition to those of the lay public, the attitudes of professionals at various levels are of concern to us [3, 5–9]. Bhugra [10] noted that we failed to educate the health professionals in addition to the relatives and friends of the mentally ill. Through direct contact with patients, through mental health education, through their students, and through interaction with policymakers their attitudes may have significant consequences. As Eker [4] noted, such information concerning definitions and attitudes of the general public and the professionals is a must to be able to decide on priorities, to understand to what extent the community services will be accepted and utilized, and to see whether there is a need for attempts to change the pattern of recognition of beliefs about and attitudes toward mental illness.

Initial Definitions of Mental Illness and Treatment Decisions

Most of the time it is the family members, friends or relatives, apart from the person himself/herself, that first become aware of the mental problem of a given person. Bhugra [10] and Mechanic [11] suggested that the early definitions of mental illness are made by primary groups within which the individual operates. If the symptoms of a person are not perceived as signs of mental illness by those close to her/him, professional help will not be accessible to the person, unless he/she is so disturbed that an outside authority intervenes. Thus, 'the basic decision about illness is usually made by community members and not professional personnel' [11, p. 27].

Quite a number of studies have been carried out about how communities define various behavioral patterns. For example, paranoid schizophrenia appears to be the behavioral pattern most widely recognized as mental illness. A study of a Nigerian sample by Erinosho and Ayonrinde [12], a Mexican-American community by Parra and Yin-Cheong So [13], Canadian nursing students by Malla and Shaw [8], and studies involving various Turkish samples (university students, nurses, patient families and relatives) by Eker [4], Arkar and Eker [2], and Eker and Arkar [6] support this conclusion. In addition, in studies compared by Roman and Floyd [14] and in various Turkish samples [2, 4, 5] the greatest social distance ratings (more rejection) were recorded for paranoid schizophrenia. This disorder was also predicted to have a poorer prognosis as compared to some other disorders [2].

As suggested by Rabkin [9], disturbed behavior that is socially visible (disruptive, bizarre, troublesome) is rejected more than withdrawn, detached or depressive behavior. The above research findings fit with the suggestion of Rabkin. Mechanic [11] suggested that mental illness becomes visible when the individual's group recognizes his/her inability and reluctance to make the proper responses in his/her network of relationships. Mechanic hypothesizes that the group tries to understand the motivation of the 'actor'. If the group members cannot empathize and understand the motivation of the actor, the likelihood of being labeled 'queer', 'strange', 'odd', or 'sick' increases. Moreover, according to Mechanic, intervention in such a situation by others is highly dependent on the visibility of the symptoms. It is when the deviancy is clearly recognized and is most disturbing to the group that various pressures are put on the person. In a similar way, Goffman [15] concluded that 'much psychotic behavior is, in the first instance, a failure to abide by rules established for the conduct of face-to-face interaction. ... Psychotic behavior is, in many instances, what might be called a situational impropriety' [p. 141].

In short, it seems that the primary groups within which the potential mentally ill operates has a significant role in the definition of illness.

Once the family and friends define the behavioral pattern of an individual as mental illness, they will intervene and search for solutions. It may be thought that in underdeveloped or developing countries where there is, on average, a lower level of education, the family, friends or the informally labeled person himself/herself may not prefer modern treatment options. Research has shown that this is not always the case. A study by Eskin [16] carried out in a rural area of Turkey did not reveal the existence of supernatural/mystical etiology of mental illness. Psychological, social and medical causes prevailed in the rural sample studied. In terms of the order of preference, the psychological etiology was the most preferred, the social the second, and the medical the third. In this same rural sample the psychiatrist was preferred as the most helpful, the mental hospital the second most helpful, and the traditional healer the least helpful source. Eskin concluded that the villagers' opinions about the causes and treatment of mental illness were similar to the conceptualizations of modern psychiatry.

Ilechukwu [17], although he did not study treatment preferences, reported that the study failed to support the frequently mentioned finding of a predominantly supernatural or mystical explanation of illness among African people. Among the psychiatric outpatients of a teaching hospital it was found that, although supernatural explanations of illness were present, mostly psychological and medical explanations were endorsed. The author predicted that if modern psychiatric approaches were more successful than traditional therapies and if modern therapies were available to most individuals, most people would use them.

In a collaborative study by the WHO [18, 19] for extending mental health care in seven developing countries, the community-based approach was emphasized. As a result of community intervention and the availability of local treatment there was an increased recognition of mentally ill individuals and an increased preference for using modern health services on the part of the community.

Although the above studies were carried out in particular samples and, therefore, the results may not generalize for a whole culture, one may predict that the availability of modern services and mental health education may result in the use of such services.

Acceptance of the Mentally Ill

As is well known by now, several research efforts have shown a generally negative and rejecting attitude on the part of the general public [9, 20–24] and an inaccurate and unfavorable presentation in the mass media [25]. Older, less educated and poorer respondents expressed less acceptance, and patients who were visibly disturbed, unpredictable, male, who belonged to a minority group, had few community ties, and were treated with somatic therapies in state hospitals elicited the most negative attitudes [26]. It seems that, once labeled, the person '... usually finds himself discriminated against in seeking to return to his old status, and on trying to find a new one in the occupational, marital, social, and other, spheres' [27, p. 87].

Cockerham [20] suggested that, although public attitudes might be becoming somewhat less negative, many former patients still lived in unpleasant circumstances because of their symptoms, lack of social support and poverty. We may have to accept the fact that, as Gralnick [28] noted, caring for the mentally ill person puts a lot of strain on his/her family. According to Gralnick if the family does not accept home care or the patient is not satisfied with his/her family, there may be a breakdown in family stability and the members may develop symptoms. We should not assume that negative attitudes are always the result of ignorance [26]. They may be due to actual past experience with a mentally ill person or to experiences communicated by others. Chakrabarti et al. [29] demonstrated that prolonged neurotic illness results in a considerable burden on the family. Wig et al. [30] noted that the mentally ill persons do have problems resulting in not living completely normal lives. Therefore, 'the community ... needs to develop a realistic, humane and sympathetic response to mental illness which takes account of the real hardships and problems faced by the mentally ill and their families' [30, p. 122].

It is at least equally important to evaluate the attitudes of the mental health professionals toward the mentally ill [3, 5–9]. The attitudes of the professionals are important due to the fact that they may have a significant impact on patients through direct contact with them or their families, through mental health education campaigns, and through contacts with policymakers. Findings show that mental health professionals may not be immune to the stereotypes of the public [3, 7, 9, 31]. In general, studies have shown that personnel with lower status have more negative attitudes than those who have advanced professional training [9]. Parallel results have been reported in Turkey by Uçman [32]. However, Rabkin [9] reported that since various categories of mental health professionals differ from each other in terms of demographic variables, such as age, sex and education, the differences in attitudes cannot be attributed solely to occupational differences.

There are studies on professionals concerning the less accepted behavioral patterns. For example, in a study involving fifth-year medical students [33] it was found that, among other findings, severity and aggressiveness of the patients' behavior was related to less acceptance. Mirabi et al. [34] showed that mental health professionals from various categories did prefer not to treat the chronic mentally ill.

Colson et al. [35], again using clinical staff from various categories, found that patient characteristics contributing to the perception of treatment difficulties were withdrawn psychoticism, severe character pathology, suicidal-depressed behavior and violence-agitation. Those perceived as improving less and having a poor prognosis were considered to be particularly difficult.

Especially in underdeveloped or developing countries there may be a need for lesser trained professionals due to inadequate number of professionals with advanced training and due to their concentration in major urban centers. Several authors have pointed out the resistance toward dealing with mental health problems among health workers in developing countries [18, 19, 36] and, in fact, in industrialized countries [1]. Beigel [1] noted that 'stigma appears to be an almost universal phenomenon. While it may assume different guises, depending on the cultural and social forces at work, fear of the mentally disordered was noted in all settings and served as a barrier to expansion of mental health care' [p. 1492].

Changing Attitudes

As it should be clear by now, if community care is to succeed, the public should be acceptant toward the mentally ill. However, we are not talking about an unrealistic level of positive attitudes. Wig et al. [30] suggested that it is wrong to impose a standardized perception. 'It does seem worthwhile, however, trying to change attitudes which are based on stigma or lack of knowledge about available treatment for the mentally ill. We are not of course attempting to induce the most favorable and optimistic view of the mentally ill imaginable' [30, p. 122].

There are a number of studies on attitude change. In her review, Rabkin [9] concluded that changes in attitudes, when they occur, after psychology courses in undergraduate samples, were probably related to variables in the teacher or in the student rather than in the course material. In studies among student nurses, hospital aides and other occupational groups, the significant factor appeared to be exposure to mental hospital and mental patients and a supplementary educational program for developing more tolerant and understanding attitudes. Bhugra [10] concluded that the effects of education on attitudes toward mental illness were mixed. Some research findings raise optimism about the effects of exposure to mental hospitals or mental patients in contributing to more tolerant attitudes in both the general public and the professionals. For example, Roman and Floyd [14] found that social acceptance was positively related to exposure to psychiatric processing systems and also that greater community optimism about the effectiveness of treatment may result from exposure to inpatient treatment systems. Using an interesting approach, Peterson [37], instead of educating the public, focused on training former patients to assume nonpatient roles. The result, as reported, was a surprising degree of community acceptance. Trute et al. [24] found that the more intimate the experience with a mentally ill, the more positive were the attitudes. Desforges et al. [38] have shown that an equal-status cooperative contact with a former mental patient resulted in attitude change among students who initially had negative attitudes, whereas merely studying in the same room did not produce any changes.

The above studies with the general public show that, in general, exposure results in more positive attitudes toward mental illness. On the other hand, there are studies which show no attitude change in the general public as a result of exposure to mental illness. For example, Sellick and Goodear [39] failed to demonstrate the influence of psychiatric exposure on public attitudes in three rural cities. A study by Arkar and Eker [2] showed that there were no differences between the attitudes of the family members who had a psychiatric patient in their families and those of a control group who had no psychiatric patients in their families. Finally, Furnham and Bower [40], in their study of lay theories of schizophrenia, reported that subjects' experience factors were not related systematically to schizophrenia questions.

Studies on professional groups have similarly resulted in inconsistent findings. We mentioned previously the conclusions of Rabkin [9] that, among health care workers, exposure and a supplementary educational program appeared to be the critical ingredient in attitude change. Jaffe et al. [41] compared student nurses who had classroom instruction only with those who had practical experience either in a 'progressive' or in a 'stereotype-supporting' mental hospital. Only the attitudes of the nurses who had practical experience in the progressive hospital changed in a more favorable direction. In a large-scale project by the WHO [19], primary health care workers in some developing countries were trained through classroom lectures and supervised experience and appreciable attitude changes toward mental illness in the health staff and the community were observed. On the other hand, Eker [3] found that, despite some significant differences, experienced clinicians were generally similar to undergraduate psychology students in their semantic differential responses.

Rabkin [42] reported similar findings in a study with a general public sample, the majority being college students, and a professional sample with postgraduate degrees. Rabkin concluded that the similarities in the views between the samples were more striking than the differences. Eker and Arkar

[6] found that, among experienced nurses each of whom worked in various fields of medicine, total years of practical experience throughout their lifetime and the number of different fields of medicine in which they worked did not predict their attitudes toward mental illness. Malla and Shaw [8], in their study comparing nursing students who were at the start of their training with those who had completed classroom instruction and experiential training, found that there were almost no differences in their attitudes. Instructional education and direct exposure to psychiatric patients did not influence most of the attitudes assessed. Finally, Arkar and Eker [5] attempted to study the influence of a 3-week psychiatric training program in medical students. Comparison of a psychiatric training group which had academic course work and practical experience with a control group in ophthalmology training revealed no differences between the groups in attitudes toward mental illness at the end of the training periods.

Both studies on the general public and those on professionals show inconsistent findings. Some support the contact hypothesis and some do not. It is difficult to give an explanation for the inconsistencies at the present state of knowledge. There may be several variables contributing to the different results. One very obvious factor is the definition of exposure. Each study has a different operationalization of the term exposure or contact. Answering questions on whether one's self, a member of one's family, or an associate had a personal experience of mental illness, whether one worked in a mental health agency as a professional or as a volunteer, interacting with a former mentally ill person under strict experimental control, or receiving various types of ongoing training programs which include various types of academic course work and practice were all utilized to study their influence on attitudes. Moreover, some studies compared mental health professionals who had various types of experiences with the public or students. Such differences in the operationalization of exposure to mental illness may be one of the significant factors contributing to inconsistent findings in the literature.

It appears that studies in this area should move to more controlled experimental designs that identify and define their variables and conditions more clearly. Two examples in this direction were reviewed above. Jaffe et al. [41] investigated the influence of training under either a 'stereotype-contradicting' or a 'stereotype-supporting' hospital and found an improvement in attitudes only in the stereotype-contradicting hospital. Desforges et al. [38] examined the influence of an equal-status cooperative contact with a former mental patient under clearly defined conditions and obtained an improvement in attitudes. More research in this direction is needed. The type of contact (e.g. formal vs. informal), the type of patient (e.g. chronicity, severity), the type of hospital environment (e.g. stereotyped vs. progressive), the duration of the contact, the content of supplementary course work, and other similar potentially significant factors should be defined and controlled in an experimental type of study. It appears that a global type of approach which does not focus on the detailed characteristics of exposure to mental illness and which assumes that being simply exposed to a mentally ill person under any type of condition is sufficient should not be expected to produce improvements in attitudes automatically.

In the research on attitude change two possibly limiting factors are the burden on the community, particularly on the family members of the mentally ill, and the public or the professionals already having optimum levels of attitudes toward the mentally ill. These factors may limit the amount of change possible under training-involving exposure. Several authors [4, 28, 30, 43] have pointed out the stress that may result from caring for the mentally ill. As mentioned above, even professionals may prefer not to work with certain types of patients [33–35] and severe cases may be difficult to manage even in the best hospital conditions [28]. Thus, as Rabkin [26] stated, present levels of attitudes may be a result of factors other than ignorance and bigotry and that we should address the balance between stigma and burden on caretakers. Moreover, Malla and Shaw [8], Eker and Arkar [6] and Arkar and Eker [5] have suggested that those choosing the health professions may already have optimum levels of attitudes and this may not leave much room for further change.

Even in the case of some general public samples, due to a relatively high educational level or due to a cultural belief system, such an optimum level may already have been reached. In general, in our studies we do not consider beforehand how much room there is for attitude change and whether that change is realistic or desirable. In fact, the existing levels may already be unrealistically optimistic as Wig et al. [30] have noted in their study.

Finally, certain types of attitudes may become fixed at a relatively early age under socialization pressures and may not be open to further change. How early various attitudes toward mental illness are formed and which of them are still open to change in a realistic direction should be addressed in future research. If particular attitudes are formed at an early age it may be necessary to educate the children at schools as early as possible about modern views on mental illness. Moreover, as Bhugra [10] suggested, 'it takes more than one generation for any change to filter through' [p. 9]. The difficulty of changing the views concerning mental illness in a society is also implied by a new concept in social psychology, namely social representations. In the following section a brief description of this concept will be made.

Social Representations

A new trend has emerged within social psychology as a critique of the orthodox attitude research. According to Moscovici [44] – the brief description of social representations given in this section is basically from this source – when social phenomena are investigated we come across explanations at the level of the individual, such as attributions, dissonance and attitudes. Attitude research is one of the approaches within social psychology that overemphasize individual representation. Therefore, Moscovici criticizes attitude research for restricting itself to an individual level of reference and for its ignorance of the collective thinking. Rather than studying the individual level of information processing, Moscovici suggests the study of social representations, their characteristic properties, the way they arise and become saturated, and the way they turn out to be our social reality. Moscovici predicts that one day social representations will replace the more traditional concepts of attitudes and opinions.

Social representations are considered as sets of concepts, statements and explanations that are created and diffused within the society. For example, a dictionary meaning of a concept or a word such as schizophrenia may have different connotations when it is socially used. Therefore, during a conversation we do not start to describe what schizophrenia means but we take certain information for granted. Social representations are loaded with unspoken information. They inform us of individuals' theories about their shared experiences and they are strengthened and changed during the course of communication. Encountered events are defined and categorized in terms of social representations. They are prescriptive in nature in that they impose themselves upon us with an irresistible force. Moscovici argues that the function of social representations is to make the unfamiliar familiar. Encountered objects and events are assigned meanings through comparisons with previous encounters, which means that social representations bring familiarity. Moreover, these familiarities are used as frames of references to define what is unfamiliar. By representing what is familiar and what is unfamiliar, social representations acquire a complementary function to that of science which turns the familiar into the unfamiliar. For example, we may already have some information about an object of study, but science renames that information by using formulas and experimental designs so that it makes the familiar unfamiliar. In order to control the possible biases, science tends to ignore social representations in creating an artificial milieu to acquire an 'objective' status of knowledge. And yet, there is always an exchange between science and social representations. As the findings of science impact upon common sense and begin to acquire the representative status of so-called 'facts', their 'representational' aspects are forgotten. They turn out to be social facts. Thus, during the course of turning what is unfamiliar into something familiar, social representations are created and they function to create and predict social reality in a continuous manner. Through social representations even science which tries to separate itself from the influence of society becomes a part of social reality.

In the light of the theory of social representations we can argue that if we are going to try to change the attitudes of professionals an common sense beliefs about mental illness, we must realize that it cannot be done in a short period of time. Long-standing new images and theories must be formed through the media so that a profound change of representations can be attained. Moreover, strengthening of social representations and changing of social representations may differ from each other in terms of degree of difficulty. Social representations are historical and widespread; therefore, it is not easy to create new representations of mental illness.

Representations of mental illness can be found in written and ordinary communications. Content analysis of the information concerning mental illness circulating in society is of central importance. After the way mental illness is represented in the media is analyzed, attempts must be made to change that representation if that is desirable. This, however, requires a considerable amount of time and consistent value targeted campaigns to create a new conscience on mental illness.

Conclusion

It seems that at the level of attitudes or social representations, a few isolated attempts in particular samples at changing them toward a more desirable direction may not be of much use. To have a widespread and long-term effect we should start early, as we suggested above, possibly at elementary school or even earlier, and use the educational system and all types of media in our attempts to change the attitudes, social representations and beliefs. We should not expect widespread changes at all levels of a society for a couple of generations and even more.

References

1   Beigel A: Community mental health care in developing countries. Am J Psychiatry 1983;140: 1491–1492.
2   Arkar H, Eker D: Influence of having a hospitalized mentally ill member in the family on attitudes toward mental patients in Turkey. Soc Psychiatry Psychiatr Epidemiol 1992;27:151–155.
3   Eker D: Attitudes of Turkish and American clinicians and Turkish psychology students towards mental patients. Int J Soc Psychiatry 1985;31:223–229.

4 Eker D: Attitudes toward mental illness: Recognition, desired social distance, expected burden and negative influence on mental health among Turkish freshmen. Soc Psychiatry Psychiatr Epidemiol 1989;24:146–150.

5 Arkar H, Eker D: Influence of a 3-week psychiatric training program on attitudes toward mental illness in medical students. Soc Psychiatry Psychiatr Epidemiol 1997;32:171–176.

6 Eker D, Arkar H: Experienced Turkish nurses' attitudes towards mental illness and the predictor variables of their attitudes. Int J Soc Psychiatry 1991;37:214–222.

7 Fryer JH, Cohen L: Effects of labeling patients 'psychiatric' or 'medical': Favorability of traits ascribed by hospital staff. Psychol Rep 1988;62:779–793.

8 Malla A, Shaw T: Attitudes towards mental illness: The influence of education and experience. Int J Soc Psychiatry 1987;33:33–41.

9 Rabkin JG: Opinions about mental illness: A review of the literature. Psychol Bull 1972;77:153–171.

10 Bhugra D: Attitudes towards mental illness: A review of the literature. Acta Psychiatr Scand 1989; 80:1–12.

11 Mechanic D: Some factors in identifying and defining mental illness; in Scheff TJ (ed): Mental Illness and Social Processes. New York, Harper, 1967, pp 23–32.

12 Erinosho OA, Ayonrinde A: A comparative study of opinion and knowledge about mental illness in different societies. Psychiatry 1978;41:403–410.

13 Parra F, Yin-Cheong So A: The changing perceptions of mental illness in a Mexican-American community. Int J Soc Psychiatry 1983;29:95–100.

14 Roman PM, Floyd HH Jr: Social acceptance of psychiatric illness and psychiatric treatment. Soc Psychiatry 1981;16:21–29.

15 Goffman E: Interaction Ritual: Essays on Face-to-Face Behavior. New York, Anchor, 1967.

16 Eskin M: Rural population's opinions about the causes of mental illness, modern psychiatric help-sources and traditional healers in Turkey. Int J Soc Psychiatry 1989;35:324–328.

17 Ilechukwu STC: Inter-relationships of beliefs about mental illness, psychiatric diagnoses and mental health care delivery among Africans. Int J Soc Psychiatry 1988;34:200–206.

18 Sartorius N, Harding TW: The WHO collaborative study on strategies for extending mental health care. I. The genesis of the study. Am J Psychiatry 1983;140:1470–1473.

19 Harding TW, d'Arrigo Busnello E, Climent CE, Diop MB, El-Hakim A, Giel R, Ibrahim HHA, Ladrido-Ignacio L, Wig NN: The WHO collaborative study on strategies for extending mental health care. III. Evaluative design and illustrative results. Am J Psychiatry 1983;140:1481–1485.

20 Cockerham WC: Sociology of Mental Disorder, ed 4. Englewood Cliffs, Prentice-Hall, 1996.

21 Greenley JR: Social factors, mental illness, and psychiatric care: Recent advances from a sociological perspective. Hosp Community Psychiatry 1984;35:813–820.

22 Rahav M, Struening EL, Andrews H: Opinions on mental illness in Israel. Soc Sci Med 1984;19: 1151–1158.

23 Socall DW, Holtgraves T: Attitudes toward the mentally ill: The effects of label and beliefs. Soc Q 1992;33:435–445.

24 Trute B, Tefft B, Segall A: Social rejection of the mentally ill: A replication study of public attitude. Soc Psychiatry Psychiatr Epidemiol 1989;24:69–76.

25 Wahl OF: Mass media images of mental illness: A review of the literature. J Community Psychol 1992;20:343–352.

26 Rabkin JG: Public attitudes: New research directions. Hosp Community Psychiatry 1981;32:157.

27 Scheff TJ: Being Mentally Ill. New York, Aldine, 1966.

28 Gralnick A: Build a better state hospital: Deinstutionalization has failed. Hosp Community Psychiatry 1985;36:738–741.

29 Chakrabarti S, Kulhara P, Verma, SK: The pattern of burden in families of neurotic patients. Soc Psychiatry Psychiatr Epidemiol 1993;28:172–177.

30 Wig NN, Suleiman MA, Routledge R, Murthy RS, Ladrido-Ignacio L, Ibrahim HHA, Harding TW: Community reactions to mental disorders: A key informant study in three developing countries. Acta Psychiatr Scand 1980;61:111–126.

31 Gutierrez JLA, Ruiz JS: A comparative study of the psychiatric nurses' attitudes towards mental patients. Int J Soc Psychiatry 1978;24:47–52.

32 Uçman P: Attitudes of psychiatric personnel and the therapeutic milieu. Hacettepe Med J 1983; 16:191–197.

33 Elizur A, Neumann M, Bawer A: Interdependency of attitudes, diagnostic assessments and therapeutic recommendations of medical students towards mental patients. Int J Soc Psychiatry 1986; 32:31–40.

34 Mirabi M, Weinman ML, Magnetti SM, Keppler KN: Professional attitudes toward the chronic mentally ill. Hosp Community Psychiatry 1985;36:404–405.

35 Colson DB, Allen JG, Coyne L, Deering D, Jehl N, Kearns W, Spohn H: Patterns of staff perception of difficult patients in a long-term psychiatric hospital. Hosp Community Psychiatry 1985;36: 168–172.

36 Murthy RS, Wig NN: The WHO collaborative study on strategies for extending mental health care. IV. A training approach to enhancing the availability of mental health manpower in a developing country. Am J Psychiatry 1983;140:1486–1490.

37 Peterson CL: Changing community attitudes toward the chronic mentally ill through a psychosocial program. Hosp Community Psychiatry 1986;37:180–182.

38 Desforges DM, Lord CG, Ramsey SL, Mason JA, Van Leeuwen MD, West SC, Lepper MR: Effects of structured cooperative contact on changing negative attitudes toward stigmatized social groups. J Pers Soc Psychol 1991;60:531–544.

39 Sellick K, Goodear J: Community attitudes toward mental illness: The influence of contact and demographic variables. Aust NZ J Psychiatry 1985;19:293–298.

40 Furnham A, Bower P: A comparison of academic and lay theories of schizophrenia. Br J Psychiatry 1992;161:201–210.

41 Jaffe Y, Maoz B, Avram L: Mental hospital experience, classroom instruction and change in conceptions and attitudes towards mental illness. Br J Med Psychol 1979;52:253–258.

42 Rabkin JG: Who is called mentally ill: Public and professional views. J Community Psychol 1979; 7:253–258.

43 Kessler RC, Price RH, Wortman CB: Social factors in psychopathology: Stress, social support, and coping processes. Annu Rev Psychol 1985;36:531–572.

44 Moscovici S: The phenomenon of social representations; in Farr R, Moscovici S (eds): Social Representations. Cambridge, CUP, 1984, pp 3–70.

Prof. Doğan Eker, Psikoloji Bölümü, O.D.T.Ü., TR–06531 Ankara (Turkey)

Guimón J, Fischer W, Sartorius N (eds): The Image of Madness. The Public Facing Mental Illness and Psychiatric Treatment. Basel, Karger, 1999, pp 13–19

....

Mental Illness as Metaphor

Asmus Finzen, Ulrike Hoffmann-Richter

Psychiatrische Universitätsklinik, Basel, Switzerland

Twenty years ago Susan Sontag published her famous essay on *Illness as Metaphor* [1]. Ten years later she wrote about *Aids and Its Metaphors* [2]. Since then it has been realized that the metaphoric use of illness and stigmatizing illness are closely connected. Metaphors of illness are widely used. All of them have one common characteristic: they imply negative or derisive connotations. Di Giacomo [3], an American ethnologist, who fell sick with leukemia while working on a research project in a hospital concludes:

> Metaphorizing cancer is invariably a process of disparagement, investing the disease with meanings that call for violent, repressive, self-righteous, even totalitarian responses.

All this is particularly true for mental illness. Mental illness as metaphor is a major complication of living with mental illness as well as of treating mental illness. Since schizophrenia, in the eyes of the public, is the prototype of mental illness, we shall illustrate this referring to schizophrenia.

Illness as Metaphor

Schizophrenia is not just the name of an illness. Mental illness and particularly schizophrenia is a metaphor, like cancer or AIDS or, in the past, tuberculosis. This metaphor is a major complication of living with mental illness as well as of treating mental illness. It is always negative, always derisive. The metaphor forwards images of acting out, violence, of incomprehensible, bizarre or contradictory behavior and thinking. The metaphoric use of schizophrenia is an important part of stigmatization, of violating the identity of those suffering from the illness called schizophrenia. The word schizophrenia is a metaphor of defamation. Its metaphoric use is an important part of stigmatization, of violating the identity of those suffering from the illness called schizophrenia [4].

The American essayist Susan Sontag has written two books on this problem. In the introduction to the first one, *Illness as Metaphor* [1], which she wrote when she was sick with cancer herself, she describes the dilemma.

She insists 'that illness is not a metaphor, and that the most truthful way of regarding illness – and the healthiest way of being ill – is one most purified of, most resistant to metaphoric thinking'.

On the other hand she admits:

Yet it is hardly possible to take up one's residence in the kingdom of the ill unprejudiced by the lurid metaphors with which it has been landscaped.

At the end of her second book, *Aids an its Metaphors* [2], she resumes:

For the time being, much in the way of individual experience and social policy depends on the struggle for rhetorical ownership of the illness: how it is possible, assimilated in argument and in cliché. The age-old, seemingly inexorable processes whereby diseases acquire meanings (by coming to stand for the deepest fears) and inflict stigma are always worth challenging, and it does seem to have more limited credibility in the modern world.

This is all the more urgent because stigmatizing certain groups of ill people is possibly not an unwanted incidence of history, but Sontag [2] suspects a basic need of society:

It seems that societies need to have one illness, which becomes identified with evil, and attaches blame to its 'victims'.

Schizophrenia, like cancer and AIDS, is apparently especially suited for this role. It is an incomprehensible and a badly understood illness. Many people experience schizophrenia as strange and frightening; and there are consequences to this way of understanding illness:

Any disease that is treated as a mystery and acutely enough feared will be felt to be morally, if not literally, contagious. Thus, a surprisingly large number of people with cancer find themselves being shunned by relatives and friends and are the object of practices of decontamination by members of their household, as if cancer, like TB, were an infectious disease. Contact with someone afflicted with a disease regarded as a mysterious malevolency inevitably feels like a trespass; worse, like the violation of a taboo. The very names of such diseases are felt to have a magic power. [1]

One can easily exchange the word cancer for the word schizophrenia in this quotation. It fits; and of course this is not without consequences.

The Terror of the Word

'Everybody who deals with psychotic patients and their families knows frightening reactions which are frequently the result of nearly mentioning the word schizophrenia. We have learned, to use it very cautiously or even not at all. Obviously the term has developed a life of its own that has nothing to do with the reality of the illness schizophrenia in present days', resumes Katschnig [5], psychiatrist in Vienna. This is not the result of failure of psychiatry in dealing with its major illness, but it is a direct consequence of the instrumentalization of the term schizophrenia as a metaphor of defamation.

Schizophrenia as a metaphor has nothing to do with the illness, the central trait of which is 'that healthy parts of personality in the schizophrenic always survive' [6]. Schizophrenia as a metaphor is always negative, always derisive. The metaphor forwards images of acting out, violence, of incomprehensible, bizarre or contradictory behavior and thinking [7–9]. In this context it does not make a difference whether teenagers think something is 'schizo', or whether politicians describe the deals of their adversaries as 'schizophrenic'. The word is an excellent way of putting rejection and contempt in just one word.

Therefore, it is not incidental that journalists and other writers who, by profession are inclined to cut things short, are especially apt to employ schizophrenia as a metaphor on many occasions. When they intend to denounce the thoughts on the acts of a person as especially contradictory or infamous they are very often called schizophrenic. They can be sure that their well-educated readers understand them; and they do: for them schizophrenia is an estrangement of mind and soul, a symbol for irrationalism, for weirdness, for unaccountability, for complete lack of responsibility. Schizophrenia as a metaphor signalizes danger. When the word schizophrenia is employed in its basic meaning as a name of an illness the metaphoric meaning is present as well and leads the stigma in a very direct way.

From *Schizogorsk* to Cultural AIDS

We shall demonstrate this with several examples. We begin with a quotation of the Swiss novelist and psychiatrist Walter Vogt, who in his novel *Schizogorsk* [10] succeeds in an especially artful interweaving of illness and metaphor:

The term of schizophrenia was introduced in 1908 or 1911 by Eugen Bleuer from Zurich. It can't be incidental that the concept of schizophrenia was developed in Switzerland and within Switzerland at Zurich. The splitting of mind and soul between puritanism and striving for work and wealth, which was condemned in the old testament, is of good protestant tradition. At Berne people would have shook their heads on absurd ideas like this and would have gone forward to state affairs. Even at Basel schizophrenia could not have been developed. The gap between the world of stiff bourgeoisie and the largest poison-kitchen in the world, this gap was much more than schizophrenia.

If we do not live in Zurich, Berne or Basel we can enjoy this subtle irony. But if even psychiatrists like Walter Vogt succumb to the temptation to use schizophrenia as a metaphor in such an infamous way, we cannot be surprised when other people do this as well; and they do it obviously joyfully and often: talkmasters like Wieland Backes and Alfred Biolek, both well known in Germany, the latter asking a member of Chancellor Kohl's cabinet: 'Don't you feel schizophrenic?'; another cabinet member, Norbert Blüm ('O holy schizophrenia'), describes the problems of the German social system in the magazine *Der Spiegel*, as many other writers in the *Frankfurter Allgemeine Zeitung*, the *Berliner Tageszeitung*, the *Hamburger Zeit* and the *Neue Zürcher Zeitung* (*NZZ*), and those of the tabloids. Among the public television chains, the official ARD is especially remarkable: it presents two cabaret shows called 'Ein Irrer ist menschlich' (crazy people are human) and another one called 'Schizofritz': crazy, isn't it?

The left wing *Berliner Tageszeitung* (*taz*) may ask for a mild judgment. One of its authors puts the word schizophrenic in an article on the occasion of the 90th birthday of Günther Anders in quotation marks: his appeal is 'schizophrenic', because political activity never is useful as Anders keeps saying.

In the *Frankfurter Allgemeine Zeitung* schizophrenia is especially frequently used in the cultural section. 'Education for schizophrenia' has been a characteristic of the former GDR education. Somebody with the initials G.R.K. states: 'The vision of the Musica universalis produces a schizophrenia on its own'. An article on theater policy in Frankfurt talks about 'one of the schizophrenias of our public support systems for theaters'. Even the economic section takes part in this game reporting on a troublesome meeting of shareholders of Lonrho: 'Shareholders: The Executive Board is Schizophrenic'.

The *Neue Zürcher Zeitung* employs the incriminating term in an almost loving way. Maybe Walter Vogt was not wrong in his insinuations on the mentality of the people of Zurich. Four times within 1 month we found metaphors of schizophrenia, e.g. a headline on 'schizophrenic drug policy' and another one 'schizophrenia without limits' referring to public measures to secure the state budget. Another headline in this context was 'schizophrenia of financial policy'. A priest is suspended after calling celibacy as 'collective schizophrenia', and the association of taxpayers considers ecological arguments for rising the prices of gasoline as 'dubious and schizophrenic'. Most of the time the paper quotes statements of third persons but obviously the editors love to quote these people when they use schizophrenia as a metaphor.

Editors and authors of the *Hamburger Zeit* seem to share the preferences of their colleagues of the *NZZ*. Hans Schüler e.g. a political editor, makes the diagnosis of 'the illness of political schizophrenia'. When we wrote to him, he ruefully promised to improve. But this is only true for him. Ulrich Greiner, a colleague, maintains in an article on the 'drug of disillusionment', this 'lifesaving schizophrenia' is intellectually not very satisfying. Another colleague seems to be keen to win the first prize in using metaphors. In an article in the Berliner *taz*, which is (most of the time) in economic difficulties he states: 'The taz planned to commit suicide.' It is 'crazily threatened'. 'What do we think about a suicidal person that asks us to stop him? Indeed: He is inclined to be schizophrenic.' The author resumes: 'This newspaper is totally crazy. We have to protect it of itself.' Who is surprised, when this paper, on the occasion of the Frankfurt Book Fair 1995, warns of 'cultural AIDS'?

Mystifying Diseases

More convincing examples for the destructive effects of the metaphoric use of illness are hardly conceivable. This is illustrated by another quotation of Susan Sontag who, in *Aids and its Metaphors* [2] reports on her own suffering experience:

Twelve years ago, when I became a cancer patient, what particularly enraged me – and distracted me from my own terror and despair at my doctors' gloomy prognosis – was seeing how much the very reputation of this illness added to the suffering of those who have it. Many fellow patients with whom I talked during my initial hospitalizations, like others I was to meet during the subsequent two and a half years that I received chemotherapy as an outpatient in several hospitals here and in France, evinced disgust at their disease and a kind of shame. They seemed to be in the grip of fantasies about their illness by which I was quite unseduced. And it occurred to me that some of these notions were the converse of now thoroughly discredited beliefs about tuberculosis.

Tuberculosis has lost its frightening power. It is no longer suitable as a metaphor of evil. As to cancer we have learned to deal with it in a more open and offensive way. Schizophrenia as a metaphor of devaluation and degradation has taken its place in many respects – as has AIDS in recent years. It may help a little, when Wing [11] reminds us that schizophrenia has nothing to do with violence at soccer games, with the behavior of stressed politicians, with drug dependence or criminal behavior or with creativity of artists or incomprehensible undertakings of managers and generals: 'It isn't even correct that all people with a diagnosis of schizophrenia are crazy; from the perspective of lay people they may seem completely healthy.'

'Mad or normal is a matter of public acceptation', Walter Vogt [12] says and the decision, if one or the other is true, is not made by psychiatrists but in the media: 'Even they don't decide themselves, they call for the decision of their readers on what they call the same judgment of the people (gesundes Volksempfinden).' The hatred of schizophrenics that became public after the assassination attempts on German politicians in 1990 underlines that Vogt is right.

Schizophrenia as a metaphor is derived from vague tragedist ideas that people have about the illness schizophrenia. The use of schizophrenia as a metaphor, in its turn, influences the public image of the illness schizophrenia and of the people suffering from schizophrenia. Since this is true we cannot be surprised that the diagnosis of schizophrenia turns out to be a second illness, an illness that has to be kept secret at any prize. When we try to understand people suffering from schizophrenia, we are hit by the terrible way in which the public image of schizophrenia augments their suffering. It distorts the way in which they see themselves, it violates their identity, and it determines the healthy deal with them in a fatal way. The ill and their families can only react by withholding information about the illness, as far as possible, and keep it in the family. As to move distant friends or people at work they better hide their illness from them.

Of course this is by no means a satisfying condition. We are called upon to denounce the metaphor of the illness and to support the ill and their families. We are called upon, as the philosopher Friedrich Nietzsche says in the *Morgenröte* [13]:

to calm the imagination of the invalid, so that at least he should not, as hitherto, have to suffer more from thinking about his illness than from the illness itself – that, I think, would be something! It would be a great deal.

We close with a last quotation from Susan Sontag about the aim of her engagement, which we share wholeheartedly:

To calm the imagination, not to incite it. Not to confer meaning, which is the traditional purpose of literary endeavor, but to deprive something of meaning: to apply that quixotic, highly polemical strategy, 'against interpretation', to the real world this time. To the body. My purpose was, above all, practical. For it was my doleful observation, repeated again and again, that the metaphoric trappings that deform the experience of having cancer have very real consequences: they inhibit people from seeking treatment early enough, or from making a greater effort to get competent treatment. The metaphors and myths, I was convinced, kill. (For instance, they make people irrationally fearful of effective measures such as chemotherapy, and foster credence in thoroughly useless remedies such as diets and psychotherapy.) I wanted to offer other people who where ill and those who care for them an instrument to dissolve these metaphors, these inhibitions. I hoped to persuade terrified people who were ill to consult doctors, or to change their incompetent doctors for competent ones, who would give them proper care. To regard cancer as if it were just a disease – a very serious one, but just a disease. Not a curse, not a punishment, not an embarrassment. Without 'meaning'. And not necessarily a death sentence (one of the mystifications is that cancer = death). *Illness as Metaphor* is not just a polemic, it is an exhortation. I was saying: Get the doctors to tell you the truth; be an informed, active patient; find yourself good treatment, because good treatment does exist (amid the widespread ineptitude). Although the remedy does not exist, more than half of all cases can be cured by existing methods of treatment.

Conclusion

Mental illness and particularly schizophrenia is a metaphor, like cancer or AIDS or, in the past, tuberculosis. This metaphor is a major complication of living with mental illness as well as of treating mental illness. It is always negative, always derisive. The metaphor forwards images of acting out, violence, of incomprehensible, bizarre or contradictory behavior and thinking. The metaphoric use of schizophrenia is an important part of stigmatization, of violating the identity of those suffering from the illness called schizophrenia.

References

1   Sontag S: Illness as Metaphor. London, Penguin Books, 1978.
2   Sontag S: Aids and Its Metaphors. London, Penguin Books, 1988.
3   Di Giacomo S: Metaphor as illness. Med Anthropol 1992;14:109–137.
4   Goffman E: Stigma. Notes on the Management of Spoiled Identity. London, Penguin Books, 1963.
5   Katschnig H: Die andere Seite der Schizophrenie. Patienten zu Hause. München, Psychologie Verlags-Union, 1977.
6   Bleuler E, Bleuler M: Lehrbuch der Schizophrenie, ed 23. Berlin, Springer, 1975.
7   Finzen A: 'Der Verwaltungsrat ist schizophren.' Die Krankheit und das Stigma. Bonn, Psychiatrie-Verlag, 1996.
8   Finzen A, Hoffmann-Richter U: Stigma and quality of life in mental disorders; in Katschnig H, Freeman H, Sartorius N (eds): Quality of Life in Mental Disorders. Chichester, Wiley, 1997.
9   Finzen A: Schizophrenie als Metapher. Psychiatr Prax 1994;21:47–49.
10 Vogt W: Schizogorsk. Zürich, Nagel & Kimche, 1977.
11 Wing JK: Innovations in social psychiatry. Psychol Med 1980;10:219–230.
12 Vogt W: Die Schizophrenie der Kunst. Eine Rede; in Kudszus W (ed): Literatur und Schizophrenie. Tübingen, Niemeyer, 1977, pp 164–175.
14 Nietzsche F: Morgenröte: Gedanken über die moralischen Vorurteile. Frankfurt a.M., Insel Verlag, 1983.

Prof. Dr. med. Asmus Finzen, Psychiatrische Universitätsklinik,
Wilhelm Klein-Strasse 27, CH–4025 Basel (Switzerland)
Tel. +41 61 325 5217, Fax +41 61 325 5582

Guimón J, Fischer W, Sartorius N (eds): The Image of Madness. The Public Facing Mental
Illness and Psychiatric Treatment. Basel, Karger, 1999, pp 20–28

....
Social Representations of Mental Illness among the Public

Matthias C. Angermeyer, Herbert Matschinger

Department of Psychiatry, University of Leipzig, Germany

The theory of social representations was formulated by Moscovici [1] with reference to Durkheim's distinction between individual and collective representations. He defines social representations as 'a system of values, beliefs and modes of action with a twofold function: first, it serves to create an order which enables individuals to orient themselves in their material and social world and to master it. Secondly, it is to facilitate communication among the members of a community by means of providing a code for naming and unequivocally classifying the various aspects of their world and of their individual history as well as that of their group' [2].

What we are dealing with here is thus social knowledge in the sense of socially created and socially shared knowledge. The study of social representations is to provide insights into the way in which a society 'thinks' with regard to a particular issue. They form the cognitive frame ('environment of thought' [3]) for our beliefs about 'reality' and shape our actions. The idea of social representations is rooted in the everyday processes of understanding and conceptualization. The focus of investigation are the processes involved in the ongoing construction of reality through the various social actors [4].

While initially, the research interest centered around the question as to how scientific theories become part of everyday knowledge, the focus has later shifted to the social construction and representation of social phenomena. Health and illness, including mental illness, are specific fields of interest in this context. Concerning the latter, one should first of all mention the study of Jodelet [5] on the lay theories of mental illness and the consequences for everyday practises resulting from them. It was carried out in a village in France, where a large proportion of the population had provided care for the mentally ill in their families for generations. Further studies on this topic can be found above all in Italy and Spain [6, 7].

In the following, we will present the results of a study on the social representation of mental illness in the German population. In the first part, we consider the question as to what the lay public associates with the word 'schizophrenia'. Our observations are based on data from a survey which we carried out in the 'new' German 'Länder' (states) in 1993. The second part of this paper deals with the question as to what the lay public believes about the causes of schizophrenia. In this connection, brief reference will be made to two other psychiatric disorders (major depression and panic disorder with agoraphobia). The results are taken from two surveys which were conducted simultaneously in the 'old' and the 'new Länder' of Germany in 1990 [8].

Associations with the Word Schizophrenia

In order to assess the spontaneous associations of the lay public with the word schizophrenia, we began our interview by asking the open-ended question. 'What is the first thing that comes to your mind if you hear the word schizophrenia?' The answers were recorded by the interviewers and later subjected to a content analysis. For that purpose, a differentiated system of categorization consisting of 54 individual categories was developed.

The five most frequently cited categories are shown in figure 1. Most frequently – in almost one third of the cases – the participants in our study first thought of a split of conscience or of personality (28.8%) or some other form of psychic split when they heard the word schizophrenia. Markedly less frequently, in only 8.8% of the cases, the occurrence of a delusion was considered characteristic for schizophrenia. 8.1% of those questioned associated schizophrenia with mental disorder, and 7.1% with nervous disorder. 4.9% connected an unfavorable course with the term schizophrenia.

The results of a study among medical students conducted at the University of Leipzig in the autumn semester 1996/1997 are interesting in this connection. Before the latter were exposed to psychiatric expert knowledge about schizophrenia as part of their studies, we asked them the same question as the general population. The tendency to associate schizophrenia with some type of a split was even stronger than in the general population. Almost two thirds of those questioned gave the respective answers. In the vast majority of the cases, explicit mention was made of a split of personality. Other types of split such as split of conscience, split of spirit or split of character were cited comparatively rarely.

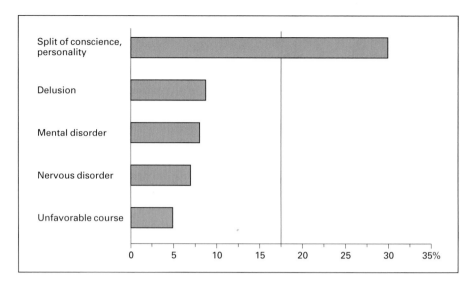

Fig. 1. The 5 most frequent associations with the word schizophrenia: general population (representative survey in the 'new' German 'Länder', 1993).

The study among medical students is particularly insightful as here, in contrast with the population survey, those questioned wrote down their ideas themselves which enabled them to provide detailed statements. Other than in the population survey where the interviewers summarized the statements of the respondents with only a few words – sometimes leaving nothing of the statement but the terse formulation 'split personality', the detailed associations of the medical students allowed us to find out more about what is actually meant by 'split'.

In principle, two fields of association can be distinguished. On the one hand, split personality signifies inconsistency, conflicting thoughts and actions, inner conflicts as well as the contrast between the conscious and the unconscious. The term thus describes a phenomenon, that, when using psychiatric terminology, one could best describe as ambivalence.

More frequently, however, a split personality is conceived of as a split into two or more personalities that exist independent of each other. Let us illustrate this interpretation with a number of quotations. Three students from Leipzig expressed their concept of schizophrenia as follows: 'Two personalities in one person, either completely or only in part, while one does not know what the other is doing. For instance, if one spends money on a new suit, the other wonders where the money has gone and where the suit comes from' – 'A person who has a number of personalities and lives these without one knowing about the existence of the other' – 'Living at two different levels of personality, without those levels being in touch and without consciousness of this situation, i.e. a person is not capable of realising that s/he lives two roles.'

It becomes apparent that the picture of schizophrenia is most frequently associated with what psychiatrists call multiple personality disorder. Regarding these results it is not surprising that four students mentioned schizophrenia and multiple personality disorder in one breath and six further students associated Dr. Jekyll and Mr. Hyde as the prototypes of a split in two personalities representing the good and the bad accordingly.

The question is now why the social representation of schizophrenia is so strongly dominated by the belief that being schizophrenic means having a split personality in the sense of a multiple personality disorder. Let us remember the history of the concept of schizophrenia: it was in 1911 that the term schizophrenia was introduced by Eugen Bleuler [9] in order to replace the name dementia praecox chosen by Emil Kraepelin. The word schizophrenia is Greek and means literally to split (schizein) and soul, mind or diaphragm (phren). At the time, Bleuler wrote: 'I call dementia praecox schizophrenia as I hope to demonstrate that the split of the various mental functions is one of its defining features.' Bleuler described schizophrenia as the loss of an integrated self, as an illness in which now this and now that psychological complex represents the personality.

From this it appears that, in the course of the popularization of Bleuler's concept of schizophrenia and its incorporation into everyday knowledge, the term was concretized as suggested by the theory of social representations. 'Tangible' persons who appear alternately and successively dominating the scene were substituted for the psychological 'complexes' which are rather difficult to grasp for the lay public (while Bleuler's concept rather implied a simultaneous 'split', see Hacking [10]). The psychological phenomena which originally 'existed' only in theory hence became concrete objects [11].

This process of concretization could also provide an explanation for the fact that medical students tended particularly strongly to connect the term schizophrenia with a split of personality. While they are likely to avail of the 'superficial knowledge' necessary to have any notion – distorted as it may be – of what could be meant more precisely by schizophrenia, many among the lay public did not know more about the disease than that it is a mental disorder.

Beliefs on the Causes of Psychiatric Disorders

As can be seen in figure 2, the most frequently reported cause of schizophrenic disorder is psychosocial stress: acute stress in the form of stressful life events and chronic stress in the form of continuous partner, family or

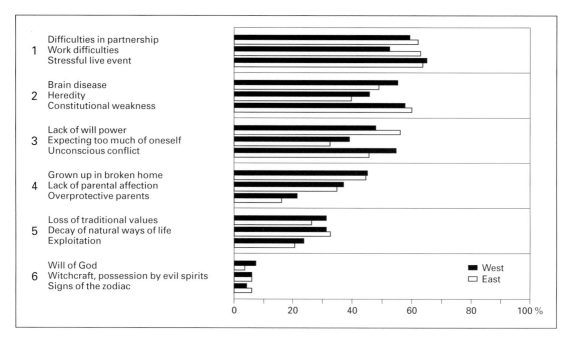

Fig. 2. Lay beliefs about the causes of schizophrenia (representative survey in the 'old' and the 'new' German 'Länder', 1990). 1 = Psychosocial stress; 2 = biological factors; 3 = intrapsychic factors; 4 = socialization; 5 = state of society; 6 = supernatural powers.

occupational stress. Respectively, more than half of those interviewed regarded these as a source of schizophrenic disorders. Second in the order of frequency are biological factors. Approximately every second person interviewed identified a brain disease or constitutional weakness as the cause of a schizophrenic disorder. Genetic factors were less often cited. Intrapsychic factors were held responsible with equivalent frequency: an unconscious conflict, lack of a strong will or, more seldom, too much ambition. Influences of socialization ranked fourth. Here the broken-home situation was regarded as etiologically relevant, followed by a lack of parental affection and overprotective parents. Only one fourth of those interviewed saw any connection with the state of society or pinpointed the destruction of natural life forms, the decay of traditional values or the exploitation of people in industrial society as causes for the occurrence of schizophrenic disorders. Only a tiny minority traces schizophrenic disorders to the influence of supernatural powers (God's will, witchcraft, possession by evil spirits, signs of the zodiac or horoscope).

This pattern was confirmed for depression and panic disorders insofar that here, too, stress was cited most frequently and supernatural powers were

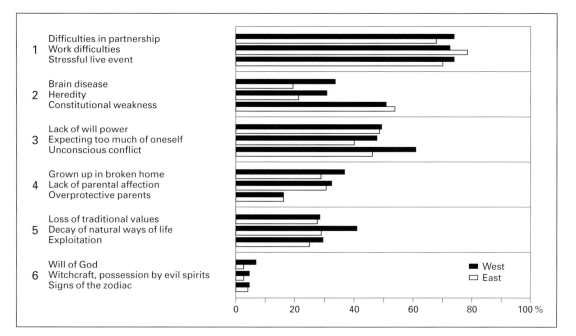

Fig. 3. Lay beliefs about the causes of major depression (representative survey in the 'old' and the 'new' German 'Länder', 1990). 1 = Psychosocial stress; 2 = biological factors; 3 = intrapsychic factors; 4 = socialization; 5 = state of society; 6 = supernatural powers.

very seldom embraced as possible causes (fig. 3, 4). In contrast with schizophrenia, intrapsychic factors ranked second and biological factors third. In line with the results regarding schizophrenic disorders, they were followed by influences of socialization and societal factors. There was no difference in the ranking order between the east and the west of Germany, disregarding the fact that with the panic disorder, those in the west assigned an etiological significance to the state of society slightly more often than to influences of socialization.

It is now important to deliberate the question as to why the concept of stress is so immensely popular with the population. Herzlich's [12] observation could provide an answer: she claims that the origins of disease are sought in the 'aggressive' society which is perceived as coercion. The latter is conveyed through the 'unhealthy way of life' in the city which is imposed by society as a burden on the individual. In the eyes of the public, illness represents social aggression. According to Herzlich, the origin of our contemporary beliefs about health and illness can be traced back to certain historical configurations and specific formations in the history of ideas: Rousseau's understanding of

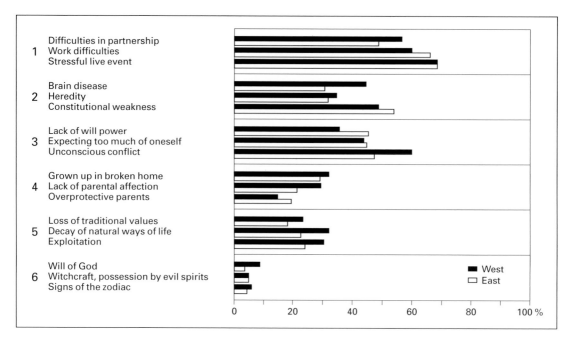

Fig. 4. Lay beliefs about the causes of panic disorder with agoraphobia (representative survey in the 'old' and the 'new' German 'Länder', 1990). 1 = Psychosocial stress; 2 = biological factors; 3 = intrapsychic factors; 4 = socialization; 5 = state of society; 6 = supernatural powers.

the relationship between man and nature, and between man and the city which had taken shape in the late 18th century. An explanation for the popularity of the concept of stress may thus lie in the fact that it fits perfectly in the critical tradition questioning the civilization process. With regard to mental illness, Srole [13] refers to the latter as the 'mental paradise lost doctrine' [p. 209]. He writes that:

Among the enduring thematic strands that weave through the long fabric of western thoughts is the conviction that contemporary man is in a condition fallen from an earlier height of simplicity, virtue and well-being. This retrospective vision harks back to the innocence of Scriptural Eden, to serenity in the Golden Age of Hellenic mythology, then to chivalric security in the medieval literature, to quintessential harmony in the Rousseauian 'state of nature', and to the earthy wholesomeness of our more recent agrarian past. Embodied in these and other variations on the same theme is a nostalgic philosophy of history, which views the complexities, heterogeneity and associated bedevilments of the present human estate as debris accumulated from the long sweep of social change.

Of those interviewed in the 'old Länder', 78.6% were indeed convinced that the extent of stress has increased within the past 20 years. Only 9.6%

thought that the level of stress had not changed. The opposite, i.e. that life had become less 'stressful', was held possible by a mere 40 of the 2,071 people questioned!

This corresponds with the result that 70.6% of those interviewed were convinced that schizophrenic disorders and depression had occurred with increasing frequency within the last 20 years. Only 12.8% were of the opinion that the prevalence of mental 'problems' had not changed. Almost nobody assumed a downward trend in the occurrence of psychiatric disorders (1.0%).

In connection with the evaluation of developments over time, it is also of interest to contrast the situation in the city with that in the country where traditional life forms are assumed to be conserved to date. It was indeed the case that the majority of the respondents (70.6%) were sure that city dwellers are more exposed to stress than people living in the country. Only 20.0% believed that living in the city or the country would not make a difference with regard to the experience of stress. A mere 33 persons could imagine that life in the country might be accompanied by more psychosocial stress than city life.

The opinion that psychiatric disorders like schizophrenia or major depression are more often observed with city residents was held by 60.2% of those questioned. Only 27.6% assumed that there was no discernible difference between urban and rural areas with regard to stress exposure.

Beside the 'good old times' whose perception is characterized by nostalgic idealization and the idyll of rural living (where time apparently stands still), the exotic regions of this planet serve as the projection screen for fantasies of 'natural' living without stress. This is particularly true for the islands of the Southern Seas, especially for Tahiti.

In the second half of the 18th century, the Southern Seas ... were discovered as a paradise on earth. In former times, the topos of the Arcadian Island, the myth of Kythera had already been part of European longings and the quintessence of utopian dreams. With Tahiti, one now believed to have found the island of freed, happy and orgiastic life. The myth of the Southern Seas was born and has not lost any of its fascination up to the present. [14, p. 19]

With this in mind, it does not come as a surprise that the majority of those interviewed was of the opinion that psychiatric disorders are more often found in the developed countries than in the developing countries. The opposite constellation was assumed by merely 4% of the respondents. 16.1% expressed the belief that first and third world countries did not differ with regard to the prevalence of psychiatric disorders.

Conclusion

In summary, we can state the following: (1) The social representation of schizophrenia is strongly shaped by the belief that the disorder involves a split of personality in the sense of a multiple personality disorder. As a possible explanation for this, a process of concretization is assumed which may have taken place in the course of the popularization of Bleuler's concept of schizophrenia and the incorporation of the latter into everyday knowledge. (2) In the majority, the lay public is of the opinion that under the living conditions of postindustrial society, we are exposed to an increasing amount of stress, that stress is *the* cause of psychiatric disorders – even those of the severity of a schizophrenic psychosis, and that the prevalence of psychiatric disorders has increased in recent times – especially in places where the process of social change has progressed particularly far.

References

1   Moscovici S: La psychanalyse, son image et son public. Paris, Presses Universitaires de France, 1961.
2   Moscovici S: Préface; in Herzlich C: Santé et maladie. Paris, Edition de l'École des Hautes Études en Sciences Sociales, 1969, pp 7–11.
3   Purkhardt SC: Transforming Social Representations. A Social Psychology of Common Sense and Science. London, Routledge, 1993.
4   Flick U: Soziale Repräsentationen in Wissen und Sprache als Zugänge zur Psychologie des Sozialen; in Flick U (ed): Psychologie des Sozialen. Reinbeck bei Hamburg, Rowohlt, 1995, pp 7–20.
5   Jodelet D: Folies et représentations sociales. Paris, Presses Universitaires de France, 1989.
6   Bellelli G: La représentation sociale de la maladie mentale. Napoli, Liguori, 1987.
7   Bellelli G: L'altra malattia. Napoli, Liguori, 1994.
8   Angermeyer MC, Matschinger H: Public attitude towards psychiatric treatment. Acta Psychiatr Scand 1996;94:326–336.
9   Bleuler E: Dementia Praecox oder die Gruppe der Schizophrenien. Leipzig, Deuticke, 1911.
10   Hacking I: Rewriting the Soul. Multipersonality and the Sciences of Memory. Princeton, Princeton University Press, 1995.
11   Sommer CM: Soziale Repräsentation und Medienkommunikation; in Flick U (ed): Psychologie des Sozialen. Reinbeck bei Hamburg, Rowohlt, 1995, pp 240–250.
12   Herzlich C: Santé et maladie: analyse d'une représentation sociale. Paris, Editions de l'Ecole des Hautes Etudes en Sciences Sociales, 1969.
13   Srole L: The Midtown Manhattan Longitudinal Study vs 'the Mental Paradise Lost' doctrine. Arch Gen Psychiatry 1980;37:209–221.
14   Pollig H: Exotische Welten. Europäische Phantasien; in Institut für Auslandsbeziehungen. Würtembergischer Kunstverein (eds): Exotische Welten. Europäische Phantasien. Stuttgart, Edition Cantz, 1987.

Prof. M.C. Angermeyer, Department of Psychiatry, University of Leipzig,
Johannisallee 20, D–04317 Leipzig (Germany)
Tel. +49 341 972 4530, Fax +49 341 972 4539

Guimón J, Fischer W, Sartorius N (eds): The Image of Madness. The Public Facing Mental Illness and Psychiatric Treatment. Basel, Karger, 1999, pp 29–37

··························

The Image of Mental Illness in Switzerland

Hans Brändli

Psychiatric Hospital, Marsens, Switzerland

It was toward the end of 1993 that the firm Lundbeck Switzerland engaged a survey institute from Zurich, the GfS, in order to analyze the extent of stigmatization of mental illness in French- and German-speaking Switzerland. This survey should have served as a base for a large-scale destigmatization campaign, hence the name 'Stigma Study Zero' [1]. A repetition of the same study was planned at the end of the destigmatization campaign. Unfortunately, it has not been possible to carry out this campaign until today, through a lack of political support and/or a lack of financial means.

Methodology

The survey had been carried out in July/August of 1994. 697 Swiss people between the ages of 18 and 84, representative of the Swiss-German and Swiss-French population, were personally interviewed, by means of a questionnaire drawn up by a group of medical directors from Swiss psychiatric institutions, including the author of this account. These medical directors were brought together by Dr. P. Spichiger-Carlsson, psychologist and author of the survey published in March 1995 [1].

Results

Around 50% of the population risk being affected, at least on one occasion, by a mental illness that necessitates professional aid from a psychiatrist or psychologist [2]. Figure 1 shows this percentage to be largely underestimated by the people interviewed.

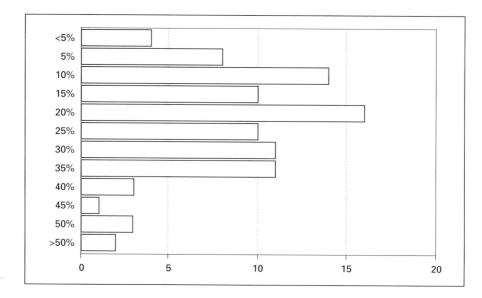

Fig. 1. Estimation of the percentage of the population who needs professional help from a psychiatrist or psychologist on at least one occasion during their lifetime; x-axis represents people interviewed (%).

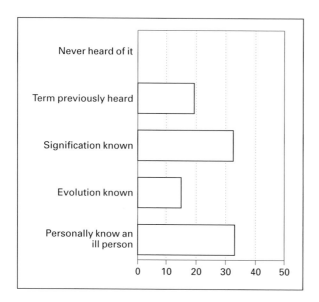

Fig. 2. Knowledge of depression (in %).

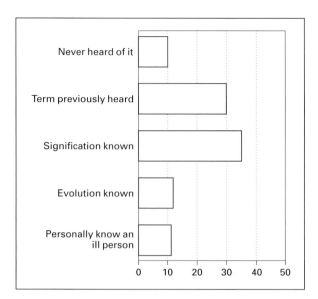

Fig. 3. Knowledge of schizophrenia (in %).

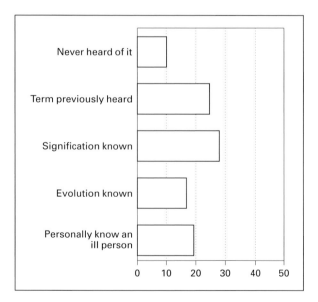

Fig. 4. Knowledge of Alzheimer's disease (in %).

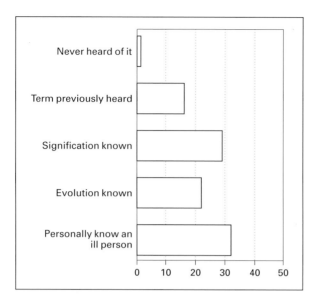

Fig. 5. Knowledge of drug addiction (in %).

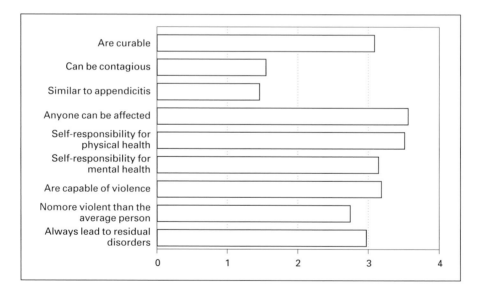

Fig. 6. Statements concerning mental illness (average). 0 = Certainly false; 4 = certainly correct.

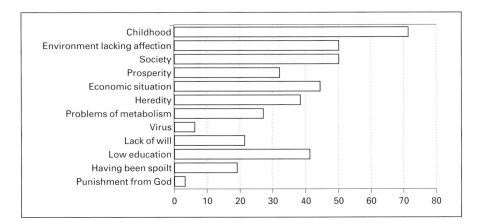

Fig. 7. Causes of mental illness (in %; multiple responses).

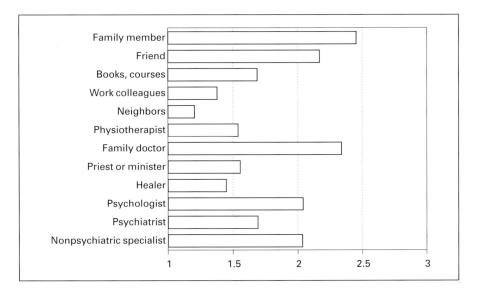

Fig. 8. Advice in cases of psychological problems: to whom would you turn? (average).
1 = Rather not; 3 = certainly.

The survey then attempted to highlight the knowledge of different mental and behavioral disorders (fig. 2–5). The relatively wide knowledge of depression is not surprising, given the frequency of this disorder. On the other hand, schizophrenia and also manic-depressive psychosis are relatively little known. The sound knowledge of Alzheimer's disease is probably due

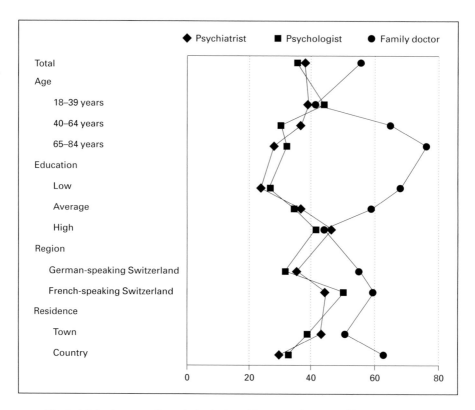

Fig. 9. Advice in cases of psychological problems: to whom would you most likely turn? (mean percentage).

to a Swiss association having operated very actively in this domain since the end of the 1980s. In Switzerland, as elsewhere in the world, the population is highly committed to the debate surrounding drug addiction, from whence comes the thorough knowledge of this subject in spite of its relatively low frequency.

Another series of questions (fig. 6, 7) aimed to better grasp false representations and prejudice. Mental illness is considered as a barely contagious affection, very different from appendicitis. On the other hand, the mentally ill person is attributed a share of self-responsibility. Figure 6 also shows the population's irrational attitude towards the mentally ill: he/she is considered as being both violent and no more violent than the average person. Despite the good prognosis attributed to mental illness, it would always provoke residual disorders. Figure 7 highlights the large responsibility bestowed upon the family of origin (childhood, low education) and upon the environment (environment

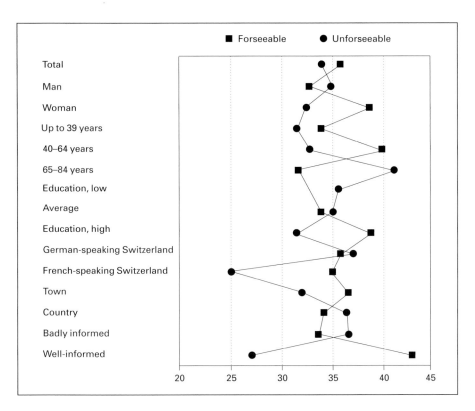

Fig. 10. Can you imagine yourself falling mentally ill and resorting to specialist help? (mean percentage).

lacking affection, society, economic situation). This contrasts with the small importance placed on heredity.

A third series of questions (fig. 8–10) were aimed at evaluating the stigma in an indirect manner. Concerning advice in the case of psychological problems (fig. 8), we were surprised by the sound reputation of the family doctor, whose advice would be sought as freely as that of the family. Whereas the help of friends is relatively frequently sought, we noted, however, a large mistrust with regard to the larger social network such as colleagues at work and neighbors. As for professionals, it is no surprise that psychologists are more easily consulted than psychiatrists. An interesting point is the high quota of appeals to nonpsychiatric specialists (surgeons, ear, nose and throat specialists, gynecologists) who were consulted for other reasons. We were expecting a greater number of appeals to ecclesiastics. We then tried to further define the relative quota of appeals to the family doctor, psychologist or psychiatrist in connection

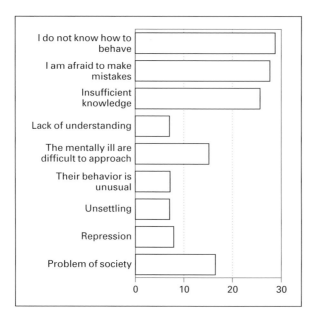

Fig. 11. Causes of problems in the approach to mentally ill patients (in %, multiple responses).

with age, education, region and residence (fig. 9). According to this breakdown, the family doctor is particularly approached by elderly people, persons of low education, and those living in the countryside. The psychologist or psychiatrist is consulted more freely by youths, people of higher education, and those living in the towns and in the French-speaking part of Switzerland. To the question, 'Can you imagine yourself falling mentally ill and resorting to specialist help?', around 1/3 replied yes, around 1/3 no (fig. 10). It is known that women more freely consult specialists than men. Regarding age, education and residence, we noted the same tendencies as in figure 9, with a marked reluctance of the German-speaking Swiss. This question was correlated with knowledge on the subject of mental illness, which proved that being well informed facilitated resorting to a specialist.

Figure 11 shows that the major difficulty in approaching a mentally ill person resides in an insufficient amount of information, making people feel incapable and fearful of making mistakes.

Conclusion

(1) Three points emerge: Stigma is closely linked to a lack of information and to prejudice. (2) Prejudice is highest among the elderly, among men, people of low education, those residing in the countryside and in the German-speaking part of Switzerland. This same population group, but without differences between regions, turns more freely to the family doctor than to a specialist in cases of psychological problems. (3) Being well informed facilitates consultation of a specialist.

References

1   Spichiger-Carlsson P: Stigmate Etudes Zéro. Zurich, Lundbeck, GfS, 1995.
2   Kessler RC, McGonagle KA, Zhao S, Nelson CB, Hughes M, Eshleman S, Wittchen HU, Kendler KS: Lifetime and 12-month prevalence of DSM-III-R psychiatric disorders in the United States. Arch Gen Psychiatry 1994;51:8–19.

Dr. Hans Brändli, Director of the Hôpital psychiatrique cantonal,
CH–1633 Marsens (Switzerland)

Guimón J, Fischer W, Sartorius N (eds): The Image of Madness. The Public Facing Mental
Illness and Psychiatric Treatment. Basel, Karger, 1999, pp 38–55

....
Public Attitudes towards Deviant Situations in Daily Life: Intervention Proposed

Danielle Goerg, Werner Fischer, Eric Zbinden, José Guimón

Department of Psychiatry, University Hospital, Geneva, Switzerland

When confronted with deviant situations in daily life, the public may perceive and interpret them in very different registers, and consider various possibilities of recourse and intervention. Questions arise as to the position medicine and, in particular, psychiatry occupy in these perceptions.

Authors like Mechanic [1] asserted, in an interactionist perspective, that if psychiatry confirms the status of the mental patient, it is generally members of the community who first noticed the existence of the disorder. Public identification of some types of deviant behavior, lay beliefs about proper intervention, possible stigmatization by the public, all play an important role in dealing with the persons manifesting such behavior.

Several studies have shown that the general public's knowledge of mental illness is often limited [2, 3]. Recognition of certain psychiatric disorders is insubstantial [4]. According to Eker [5] in a student survey, Eker and Arkar [6] in a survey of nurses, Arkar and Eker [7] in a population having a close connection with someone hospitalized for a somatic or a psychiatric illness, paranoid schizophrenia is the disorder which is, relatively, the most frequently identified. Other disorders are even less well known or fewer differentiations are made. The spectrum seems sometimes reduced, in the general public, to two extremes: madness, on the one hand, and, on the other, psychological disorders, a category into which the public places certain serious problems, such as clinical depression [8]. Public conceptions of the etiology of mental disorders, their prognosis and their treatment are often far from the current state of the psychiatric art. Thus, psychosocial stress predominates in the social representation of the causes of schizophrenia in the German public [9].

Among the various forms of help considered by the public in two regions of Great Britain, studied by Hall et al. [4], advice from a friend ranks first. Mention of a psychiatrist follows, then the family doctor. People from Quebec, interviewed by Lamontagne [2], would advise, in cases of mental health problems, to seek the assistance first of the physician, then the psychiatrist, the psychologist or some other therapist. Finally, with regard to treatment, the public favors markedly, in its beliefs and representations, the use of psychotherapy. It also considers favorably some forms of treatment such as relaxation techniques, meditation or yoga, natural medicines, and it only much more rarely takes into consideration pharmacotherapy [8, 10, 11].

The literature quoted used, in order to outline public opinion, descriptions of clinical cases, either vignettes or brief summaries, highlighting one or more of the principal symptoms of a psychiatric disorder. The underlying perspective is always that of the relationship of lay knowledge, beliefs and representation to current psychiatric categories and science.

In opposition to this psychiatric approach, the perspective chosen here favors the social environment in which various deviant behaviors are observed. Thus instances of behavior deemed inappropriate were mentioned, but with no reference to psychiatric nosography: withdrawal, agitation, bizarre or violent behavior.

The objective is to discern the public representation of some deviant behavior in everyday life and, more specifically, to learn what solutions the public proposes relative to possible intervention or persons who can be called upon. Social representations are defined, following the studies of Moscovici [12], and Herzlich [13], as notions of 'common knowledge', practical concepts that are socially created and socially shared [14]. Taking into consideration the importance of medicine and psychiatry in the definition of disorders, we are particularly interested in medical and psychiatric treatment. And it is public perception of psychiatry which will be most specifically studied. Psychiatry fulfils several functions. It can be presumed that, according to their social background, their career and their experience, social subjects would have different representations of deviancy, how it should be dealt with and, therefore, what the mandate of psychiatry is. On one hand, little differentiation in disorders and treatment might be related to the controlling functions of psychiatry and, on the other, more differentiated social representations of disorders and treatment might correspond more closely to classic psychiatry.

The three following questions will thus be examined: (1) When confronted with situations involving deviant behavior, does the public envisage similar forms of intervention or intervention differentiated according to the situation? (2) Does the public give preference to certain forms of intervention and, if so, to which ones? (3) What are the characteristics of members of the public who prefer certain forms of intervention?

Material and Methods

These questions were asked within the framework of a study carried out of public attitudes towards psychiatric treatment and psychotropic medication. The survey was undertaken in Geneva, in 1996, on a representative sample of 324 persons aged between 20 and 75 years. A questionnaire, containing both open-ended and closed questions, was used in the interviews.

In order to better discern the attitudes of interview subjects towards manifestations of deviant behavior, examples that can be encountered in everyday life were described. For each of the four types of deviant behavior – bizarre conduct, agitation, violence and withdrawal, two typical situations were described, one in public, the other in private. Certain studies, such as those of Goffman [15], show that the identification of the disorder, the handling of it and its stigmatization do not occur in the same way according to whether the behavior occurs in public or private. Overall 8 scenarios were presented (see Appendix). As an example, situations were described such as 'someone talking aloud to him- or herself or screaming in the street' or 'someone who shuts him- or herself away, never goes out, draws the curtains or closes the shutters and refuses to see anyone'. If these behaviors are defined in social terms, they may, however, also form part of a description of persons requiring psychiatric treatment.

Subjects had to choose, out of a list of forms of intervention or of persons called upon to intervene, what would be most helpful for the person concerned to cope with his or her situation: recourse to a physician, a psychiatrist, a psychologist or a trusted confidant, as well as the use of drugs – drugs in general and those specifically designed to treat mental disorders, natural medicine, rest, or finally, the choice of doing nothing. For each situation, interviewees were offered up to three possible solutions. Since natural medicine and rest did not figure as solutions to violent behavior, they will, therefore, not be examined here. Any mention of psychotropic drugs and drugs in general were regrouped, as there were few answers. Finally, it must be noted that, faced with deviant behavior, various persons were proposed, taken particularly from the medical or psychological worlds. Others, belonging to social services or the judiciary, could also have been chosen, and the relative ranks of the therapists examined might have been slightly different.

In addition to deviant situations, the questionnaire investigated various dimensions which could be linked to them. These mainly dealt with representations of mental illness (etiology, likely treatment, prognosis) by using three clinical vignettes, attitudes towards the mentally ill (scale by Cohen and Struening [16], modified), attitudes towards psychiatric medication (scale used by Guimón et al. [17]) and towards drugs in general. Also taken into consideration were prior familiarity with psychiatry (knowledge of institutions or persons working in this field, for example), experience subjects might have had, directly or within their environment, with psychiatric disorders and psychological or psychiatric treatment. The social, professional and cultural characteristics of the subjects were also examined.

Insofar as statistical methods are concerned, for attitudes with regard to the mentally ill, psychotropic medication and medication in general, factor analyses were carried out and indices (cumulative scores) created taking into account variables which saturate factors at more than 0.40. For other data (information on psychiatry, contacts with psychiatry, experiences of mental disorders), indices were established in order to synthesize data from several variables.

In order to compare answer profiles for the different scenarios, proximity measures (correlations, coefficients of dissimilarity) were used. The χ^2 test was used to compare dichotomic or dichotomized variables, the Mann-Whitney test for ordinal variables.

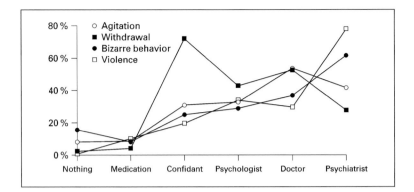

Fig. 1. Proposed intervention according to types of behavior.

Results

Differentiation in Forms of Intervention according to the Situation

The question arises, when faced with manifestations of deviant behavior, if the public envisages similar solutions or solutions differentiated according to the situation. As the two situations highlighting the same type of behavior gave rise to very similar answers, particularly concerning violence (correlation 0.97), bizarre behavior (0.94), withdrawal (0.85), slightly less for agitation (0.56), it was decided that these examples be grouped together. It is sufficient for an answer to be mentioned in one of the two situations for it to be cited. This result seems to weaken the hypothesis of the specific response to the behavior described, depending on whether it is manifested in public or in private.

Contrasted answer profiles correspond to the four types of grouped behaviors (fig. 1). If certain similarities do exist between the answers given at the description of violent or bizarre behavior, slightly fewer exist for agitation, and all three are distinguished distinctly from the answers on withdrawal. In relation to forms of intervention mentioned by subjects, it is noted that medication is relegated to a marginal position, as only 4–10% of subjects suggested it, depending on the type of behavior.

Two categories of therapists play a relatively important role: the physician and the psychologist. The physician is named by 29% of subjects in cases of violent behavior, by 37% for bizarre conduct, and by more than half for withdrawal or agitation (53%). Recourse to a psychologist is mentioned by approximately a third of interviewees in instances of bizarre behavior (29%), agitation (33%) and violence (34%), and by 43% for withdrawal symptoms. The roles of these two therapists do not appear to be very specific, as they

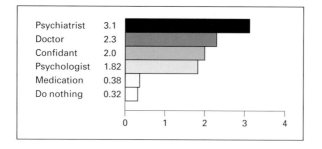

Psychiatrist	3.1	
Doctor	2.3	
Confidant	2.0	
Psychologist	1.82	
Medication	0.38	
Do nothing	0.32	

Fig. 2. Proposed forms of intervention: mean number of mentions; x-axis represents number of scenarios.

are mentioned by one third to more than one half of subjects, for the four types of behavior.

The most distinctly contrasted answers concern the psychiatrist and the confidant. Recourse to a psychiatrist is most frequently mentioned in cases of violence – by 77% of subjects, followed by bizarre conduct (61%), then agitation (41%). However, the idea of contacting a psychiatrist is rarely mentioned for withdrawal, since only 28% of subjects considered it appropriate. With regard to withdrawal, being able to talk to someone in whom the person has confidence, is very strongly the public's choice (72%), while this solution is rarely put forward for the three other types of behavior (agitation 31%, bizarre conduct 25%, violence 20%). Recourse to a psychiatrist seems, therefore, linked to socially visible behavior which may be disturbing. In contrast, the possible severity of signs of withdrawal, which psychiatrists would undoubtedly be concerned about, seems to be underestimated by the public.

Favored Forms of Intervention

If not only the four types of grouped behaviors, but also the entirety of the eight situations described are taken into account, what intervention does the public favor? In order to evaluate the relative importance of the various forms of intervention, we added, for each, the number of times an interviewee mentioned it for the 8 scenarios. We then obtained, for each intervention, an index ranging from 0 to 8.

The average number of answers varies greatly (fig. 2). More clearly than what was observed in answer profiles, it is the psychiatrist who is most frequently mentioned. He or she is named, on average, in more than 3 scenarios out of 8. The psychiatrist's role in relation to deviant behavior appears thus to be very important. The psychiatrist is followed by the physician, a confidant, then the psychologist. Medication is very rarely mentioned. The scarce suggestion of medication can be compared to results of other studies undertaken with a more direct psychiatric approach [8, 10, 11]. The various scenarios described gave rise to few multiple answers. Three answers were possible, but single answers predominated, the average per situation being between 1.1 and 1.6. It was for situations displaying withdrawal symptoms that interviewees gave the greatest number of answers.

Forms of Intervention and Characteristics of the Subjects

It might be assumed that interviewees would favor a given form of intervention according to their own social characteristics, their integration or their past experience with psychiatry. Furthermore, their preferences with regard to forms of intervention are undoubtedly not isolated from their overall representations and attitudes. Therefore, what is interesting here are the factors determining choices expressed, and the attitudes, representations and beliefs in whose context the suggestions were made. The categories of persons most frequently selected are examined: the confidant, the psychologist, the physician and the psychiatrist.

We present only the attributes which differentiate, in a statistically significant way, the subjects who chose the considered intervention very frequently from those who did not (χ^2 for dichotomic or dichotomized variables; Mann-Whitney for ordinal variables). It is considered that a form of intervention is frequently mentioned if it is named in at least four out of the eight situations described. It is rarely mentioned if it is not named, or named only once. The intermediate category has been set aside in this comparison. Concerning recourse to a psychiatrist, another approach was chosen, details of which will be given later.

Well-Informed and Competent Lay Counsellors

The idea of frequently requesting help from a confidant received relatively little support from the general public, as only 16% of subjects interviewed named it; 42% never, or rarely, did. This is, however, related to certain particularities (table 1).

As we just mentioned, in table 1 as in all the others, a selection of variables was done. The mention of the attributes which characterize the category of persons who most frequently chose a form of intervention implies a lower incidence, or the absence of, these attributes in the category of subjects who never, or only rarely, proposed this form of intervention.

Subjects who conceive of recourse to a confidant come from higher socio-professional classes (white-collar workers, members of trained or professional groups). Having always lived in Geneva or having moved here long ago, they are culturally well integrated into the community. They themselves, or their

Table 1. Well-informed lay counsellors

Variables	Attributes of category of persons
Deviant situations: alternative forms of intervention proposed	+physician* −psychiatrist***
Etiology of psychiatric disorders	+psychological factors*
Attitudes towards the mentally ill	−authoritarian* −incriminations about personal and family responsibility***
Attitudes in the subject's environment towards medication	+distrust*
Proximity to/contact with psychiatry	+information about mental illness** +contacts with institutions or persons working in psychiatry** +personal experience or experience within the subject's environment of mental disorder*
Social, professional and cultural background	+socioprofessional level – medium to high* +activities in health, social or educational fields* +residence in Geneva: native or long-term*

Characteristics differentiating subjects having frequently suggested recourse to a confidant (15.7% of the total) from those who never, or only rarely, mentioned it (42.0%). The orientations of the relationship is indicated by + or −. *$p < 0.05$; **$p < 0.01$; ***$p < 0.001$.

families, often work in fields that may have certain affinities with psychiatry, such as health care, education, social services or humanitarian activities. Their experience of the psychiatric world is relatively differentiated. Through various media, like newspapers, television and specialized literature, they have, in fact, become well informed about psychiatry. They are familiar with psychiatric institutions or know people working in them. Finally, they themselves or those close to them may have had mental problems and may even have undergone psychological or psychiatric treatment.

In the views they have of the etiology of mental disorders, these subjects underline the importance of psychological factors (personal psychological problems, lack of willpower, too demanding of themselves). And in their attitudes towards psychiatric patients, as measured on the scale of Cohen and Struening [16], they manifest little authoritarianism and do not think that patients themselves, or their families, are the cause of their mental disorders.

For them, recourse to a confidant might be envisaged as a first step, with a further suggestion that a physician be consulted, even though their family expresses misgivings with regard to medication. In contrast, they seem to exclude consulting a psychiatrist. In general, favoring advice from a friend is usually presented in direct opposition to psychiatric intervention (correlation −0.317; p < 0.01).

Thus, contrary to expectations, subjects who most frequently chose to rely on a confidant did so despite their knowledge of alternatives. This choice is doubtless the reflection of the self-confidence engendered by their social status, their social integration and a certain knowledge of the field. Indirectly, we detect the emergence of the social representation of well-informed and competent lay counsellors.

Psychological Assistance

The option of frequently consulting a psychologist was chosen by only 18% of interviewees. If these subjects resemble, in certain aspects, those who chose recourse to a confidant – the absence of authoritarian attitudes towards the mentally ill, well-informed about mental illness, contacts with fields linked to psychiatry, cultural integration, they are clearly differentiated by other aspects (table 2). When faced with descriptions of deviant situations, they reject the idea of consulting a physician and are reticent about the use of drugs, whose effectiveness they doubt in any case. For a clinical case, they suggest, in a very coherent way, the use of psychotherapy. And they also consider yoga or meditation.

Regarding the etiology of psychiatric disorders, they particularly point to the weight of factors linked to socialization (lack of affection from parents, separation from parents during childhood, overprotective parents). In contrast, they exclude other factors, be they biological (diseases of the brain, constitutional weakness, heredity), psychosocial (important events, difficulties at work, family or marital problems), societal (social inequalities, disappearance of traditional values, living conditions that are not in harmony with nature) or the supernatural (the will of God, astrology, witchcraft). They did not express socially restricting attitudes towards the mentally ill.

These subjects were distinguished, in their social background, by the fact that they tended to be younger, and their lifestyles less traditional than those either living alone or with a partner.

Common Medical Assistance

More than a quarter (28%) of the public frequently suggests consulting a physician. This preference for a physician is not socially profiled, in contrast to what has already been seen with respect to the choice of a confidant and,

Table 2. Psychological assistance

Variables	Attributes of category of persons
Deviant situations: alternative forms of intervention proposed	−physician* −medication*
Treatment of psychiatric disorders	+individual psychotherapy*** +meditation, yoga***
Etiology of psychiatric disorders	+socialization factors* −biological factors** −psychosocial factors** −societal factors* −supernatural factors*
Attitudes towards the mentally ill	−authoritarian* −social restrictions*
Attitudes towards medication in general	−effectiveness of medication*
Proximity to/contact with psychiatry	+information about mental illness*
Social, professional and cultural background	+youth** −living alone or with partner with or without children* −cultural differentiation*** +activities in health, social or educational fields***

Characteristics differentiating subjects having frequently mentioned consulting a psychologist (18.2%) from subjects who never, or rarely, mentioned it (52.5%). For further explanations, see footnote to table 1.

although less, to psychological assistance. No social characteristic clearly distinguishes these subjects, who may be familiar with psychiatric institutions or know persons working in the field of psychiatry or psychology (table 3). This preference forms part of a system of attitudes or beliefs which can be characterized as showing more tolerance or understanding towards psychiatric patients, even while displaying more reticence towards specialists in the field.

Presented with deviant behavior situations, these subjects also chose to contact a confidant, but they did not suggest consulting a psychologist or a psychiatrist. In their attitudes towards psychiatric patients, they show particular kindness and they do not blame the patient or his or her family for causing the psychiatric disorder. Finally, with respect to their attitudes towards

Table 3. Common medical assistance

Variables	Attributes of category of persons
Deviant situations: alternative forms of intervention proposed	+confidant* −psychologist* −psychiatrist*
Attitudes towards the mentally ill	+sympathetic* −incriminations about personal family responsibility**
Attitudes towards psychiatric medication	−blaming society for drug consumption***
Attitudes towards medication in general	−moral judgment on drug consumption*
Proximity to/contact with psychiatry	+familiarity with institutions or contacts with persons working in psychiatry**

Characteristics differentiating subjects having frequently mentioned consulting a physician (28.4%) from subjects who never, or rarely, mentioned it (44.1%). For further explanations, see footnote to table 1.

psychotropic medication (measured on the scale of Guimón and Ozamis [17]), they did not blame society for drug consumption and they did not make moral judgments about drug use.

It is doubtless the fairly banal image of the family doctor or the consulting physician which appears here, a doctor to whom, in a very general manner, responsibility is delegated for handling the disorder and deviant behavior, and the underlying representation is that of common or everyday medical assistance.

Specialized Psychiatric Assistance

The possibility of consulting a psychiatrist when faced with descriptions of deviant situations is, as we have seen, very often considered by the public. For 43% of all subjects, such a recourse is even frequently taken into consideration.

Now it could well be that frequent recourse to a psychiatrist is chosen by two different categories of subjects, one having a certain familiarity with, or even a close proximity to, psychiatry or mental disorders, either personally or within their environment, and the other who has no, or very little, experience. In order to distinguish the two categories, two indices were taken into account. The first one is an overall index of proximity to psychiatry, which measures the geographic or social closeness to psychiatry and the existence of relationships with people working in this field. The second is an overall index of experience, which indicates the knowledge that the subject has of psychiatric disorders or psychological or psychiatric treatment, either personally or among close or more distant relations. Those who obtain higher scores on both indices (above average) are considered to have considerable knowledge of psychiatry; they represent 33% of the subjects who frequently suggested consulting a psychiatrist. Those who, while frequently mentioning the psychiatrist, have lower scores on both indices are considered to have a negligible knowledge of psychiatry (41%). The others (26%) have average knowledge. We have compared here the subjects belonging to one of the extreme categories to the total of those belonging to the opposite category and to the medium category.

The subjects who had considerable knowledge of psychiatry, as it has just been defined, were also those who worked, themselves or someone close to them, in the fields of education, social work, health care, humanitarian activities, who take part in associations connected to these fields, and who are well informed about mental illness.

Qualified Psychiatric Assistance. The subjects who very frequently chose recourse to a psychiatrist, and who have considerable knowledge of psychiatry, were also favorable to consulting a physician when presented with cases of deviant behavior (table 4). Confronted with a clinical case study, they suggested individual psychotherapy as well as medication. They did not make any moral judgments on the consumption of drugs in general. In their attitudes towards the mentally ill, they were rarely authoritarian. These subjects, whom we consider presenting an enlightened view of psychiatry, are mainly white-collar workers, trained or professional staff. Their educational backgrounds were not manual work and ranged up to university level, sometimes in social work or medical fields.

Undifferentiated Psychiatric Recourse. An entirely different assessment can be made of those subjects who, while frequently delegating responsibility to a psychiatrist when faced with deviant behavior, have no experience of the psychiatric domain. In relation to deviant situations, they do not believe that confiding in a trusted friend or relative is useful. Questioned about the treatment necessary for a clinical case, they exclude the idea of medication, to which they attribute negative side effects. In their attitudes towards psychiatric patients, they are alone in blaming the patient and the family for causing the disorder. This explains no doubt their retaining, in the etiology of the disorders, factors linked to socialization, as defenders of psychological recourse, but probably in a very different sense.

These subjects, who are most often men, present some social status inconsistencies. They live more rarely with a partner or children. More frequently,

Table 4. Specialized psychiatric assistance

	Subjects with knowledge of psychiatry	
	important (n = 45)	negligible (n = 57)
Deviant situations: alternative forms of intervention proposed	+ physician* + medication*	− confidant**
Etiology of psychiatric disorders		− psychological factors* − socialization factors*
Treatment of psychiatric disorders	+ psychotherapy* + medication**	− medication*
Attitudes towards the mentally ill		+ personal and familial blame**
Attitudes towards psychiatric medication		+ negative side effects of drugs*
Attitudes towards medication in general	− moral judgment on drug consumption**	
Social, professional and cultural background		+ men* − familial integration* − cultural integration*
	+ nonmanual training, social, health, university*	+ no training, or manual, technical, commercial***
	+ white-collar, trained or professional staff **	+ workers, self-employed**
		+ politically right-wing*

For further explanations, see footnote to table 1.

they moved to Geneva, rather than having been born here; they are not well integrated culturally speaking. They have no training or, if they do, it is mainly in manual tasks or in the technical or commercial areas. They are currently employed either as workers or are self-employed in small businesses, and it is well known that these economic sectors are currently undergoing pronounced difficulties. Finally, these subjects were also the only ones who, in the views they expressed, were on the right-wing of the political spectrum.

Thus it appears that two categories of subjects, presenting very different characteristics as much in their social and cultural attributes as in their attitudes and representations, consider frequent recourse to psychiatric help as being pertinent.

Discussion

Differentiation of the Situations

Faced with various scenarios describing deviant behavior such as it might be noticed in daily life, the public proposes different forms of intervention. Now, indirectly, the forms of intervention suggested allow us to better interpret the social representation the public has of the different situations. In certain situations, recourse to a confidant is preferred; in others, referral to a psychiatrist predominates, while the proposal of seeking help from a physician or a psychologist is less dependent on the situation. The idea of seeking advice from a nonspecialized nonprofessional is expressed above all in situations where withdrawal signs are portrayed. In contrast, the suggestion of calling upon specialized psychiatric assistance is much more frequent in situations of violence and bizarre conduct, as well as in those of agitation, but to a lesser degree.

It would thus appear that the public representations of deviant situations are schematically structured along two axes: one mainly concerned with situations of violence and bizarre behavior, the other with withdrawal. These two axes present a certain analogy with the results of several studies realized in a more clinical perspective, through the use of vignettes or brief descriptions of the principal symptoms of certain mental illnesses. Paranoid schizophrenia is viewed, on the one hand, within a context of illness or even madness and, on the other hand, there is a whole series of diagnoses which may, like depression, not be perceived by the public as being illnesses [5–8, 10]. Despite the different approaches, it is therefore suggested that the same underlying structure exists for both representations.

Coherence of the Representations

The forms of intervention proposed correspond, for the subjects, to other representations and attitudes, and there is a tendency to include these in more general attitudes. Thus, the subjects who frequently proposed calling upon a psychologist in deviant situations also rejected consulting a physician and the use of medication. Confronted with a clinical case study, presented as a vignette, they recommended psychotherapy. With regard to their beliefs concerning the etiology of mental illness, they underlined the importance of childhood experiences and particularly those factors linked to the parent-child relationship. In contrast, they tended to exclude biological or social causes. It is very clearly a psychological point of view which emerges in this instance and it runs in parallel with attitudes which are unrestricting towards mental patients.

The idea of consulting a physician, a recourse which is much less specific, is included in an altruistic and sympathetic mind: advice from a confidant is suggested, attitudes towards psychiatric patients are tolerant, no blame is placed on patients or their families and the use of drugs is not censured.

With respect to psychiatric help, we have seen that it can be included in two different representation and attitude configurations. With regard to subjects having a certain familiarity with psychiatry, recourse to a psychiatrist corresponds to an image that can be termed medicopsychiatric. The consulting physician is also mentioned and treatment, be it pharmacological or psychotherapeutic, is considered to be appropriate. In contrast, in the absence of any knowledge of psychiatry, the idea of consulting a psychiatrist corresponds to more suspicious, distrustful or negative attitudes: asking advice of a confidant, like medication, does not appear pertinent, and blame appears to be placed on patients or their families for causing the disorder. These different examples show that the preference for a certain type of intervention takes root in the more general representations and attitudes of the subjects interviewed.

Differentiation in Social Connotations of the Forms of Intervention

If the suggestions made by the subjects showing a preference for certain particular forms of intervention can be interpreted within the context of other orientations, they may also refer back to differences in social integration and various social experiences. Even if this is not the case for common medical assistance, which has not been profiled in a social context and which is valid for the public as a whole, the other references tend to be mentioned by subjects presenting distinct characteristics and experiences. Thus, the idea of calling upon a psychologist is the prerogative of younger subjects, well assimilated into the culture, often working in a field with some connection to psychiatry and well informed about it. Requesting help from a lay person – especially suggested for cases of withdrawal, i.e. for situations that are not obvious and that do not create social disturbance – is preferred by subjects belonging to the middle to upper classes, culturally assimilated, who have personal contacts with psychiatry and are well informed about it. They clearly exclude, however, the option of consulting a psychiatrist.

Now, a proportion of the subjects who chose recourse to a psychiatrist, resemble, in numerous aspects, those who prefer asking advice from a confidant (social class, closeness to the world of psychiatry). It would, therefore, be important to determine what other factors, what other experiences, cause such opposing representations of possible sources of help. Our study does not allow us to pursue this subject in more depth.

A reference to psychiatry could also be considered by subjects who had no ties to this field in their cultural and social integration (which were often difficult or precarious), and who lacked knowledge of psychiatry or any contact with it. This brings up the question of the relationship of the public with psychiatry.

The Relationship with Psychiatry

The importance of consulting a psychiatrist in deviant situations receives considerable support, even more so in cases with elements of violence or bizarre behavior, while signs of withdrawal evoke far less often the idea of psychiatric intervention.

The logic behind consulting a psychiatrist and, therefore – indirectly – the image the public has of him or her, is twofold corresponding to the different functions of psychiatry. This recourse can be interpreted in a social control perspective. It is the idea of reestablishing a perturbed social order by simply delegating the problem to psychiatry, with no knowledge of the means at its disposal. The subjects who were most marginalized socially, culturally and in their experience of psychiatry were the holders of these representations. This recourse can also be interpreted within an overall care framework. Various forms of treatment are proposed, ranging from medication to psychotherapy, and different therapists, mainly the physician, are mentioned. This image of the psychiatrist is that preferred by subjects who are well integrated in society and who may have had some experience with psychiatry. Hall et al. [4] observed that, if more educated subjects suggested a greater number of sources of assistance, recourse to a psychiatrist was particularly chosen by those coming from a higher social class and with a background of higher education, and by women.

It must be pointed out that the importance attributed to various specialists such as physicians, psychologists and psychiatrists must, however, be placed within the urban context of this study. Geneva, an urban center, whose population, in the great majority, works in the service sector, has a very high physician-to-inhabitant ratio. Its institutional and private psychiatric services are very well developed. A large number of psychologists work both in public social services and in private practices. The use of medical, psychiatric or psychological therapy is particularly great. It may, therefore, be assumed that the general public is very familiar with popular notions of medicine or psychology.

Certain results of our study give evidence as to how widespread these perceptions are. We have noted that the idea of consulting a psychologist is part of an overall psychological viewpoint, mainly held by younger subjects. It is they who have been influenced most by the pervasiveness of psychology in the pop culture. The priority given by the public to psychiatry when confronted with deviant situations also appears higher than in certain other studies, though a rigorous comparison is not possible, since the approach of those studies is more clinical and the persons proposed sometimes different. It was noted, however, that people from Quebec, in cases of mental illness, prefer consulting a physician to a psychiatrist, psychologist or other therapist [2]. In the two communities surveyed by Hall et al. [4] in Great Britain, the idea of asking advice from a friend has priority over consulting a psychiatrist for all the clinical scenarios (depression, obsessional neurosis and schizophrenic defect state) with the exception of paranoid schizophrenia. In a study conducted in Germany [8], it is only in cases of schizophrenia that more than half those interviewed (57%) suggested a psychiatrist: in the case of compulsive disorders only one third, approximately a fourth in the case of manic episodes, and even less for other clinical cases described. Therefore, it would be important to study, within varying geographic and social contexts, the public image of the different persons who may be called upon to intervene in situations of deviant behavior or manifestations of mental disorder.

Conclusion

Public attitudes towards psychiatric treatment and psychotropic medication were studied in a survey carried out in Geneva on a representative sample of 324 persons aged between 20 and 75. Confronted with the description of deviant situations that can be encountered in daily life, the public first considers recourse to a psychiatrist, whose role in relation to deviant behavior thus appears to be very important. Help from a physician, a confidant or a psychologist is also envisaged. Medication is very rarely mentioned. Preference for a certain type of intervention takes root in the more general representations and attitudes of the subjects interviewed and is often linked to their social and cultural characteristics.

Recourse to a psychiatrist is linked to socially visible behavior which may be disturbing. In contrast, the possible severity of signs of withdrawal, which psychiatrists would undoubtedly be concerned about, is underestimated by the public. Two categories of subjects, presenting very different characteristics in their social and cultural attributes and in their attitudes and representations, consider frequent recourse to psychiatric help to be pertinent.

If recourse to a physician is rather unspecific, choosing to rely on a confidant seems to reflect the self-confidence engendered by higher social status, social integration and a certain knowledge of the field. People considering psychological help do not express socially restricting attitudes towards the mentally ill. In the etiology of psychiatric disorders they particularly point to the weight of factors linked to socialization (lack of affection from parents) and they exclude other factors, be they biological, psychosocial or supernatural.

Appendix

Deviant Situations

Agitation
Someone who, in a movie theater, cannot sit still, fidgets, gets up and sits down repeatedly and talks incessantly.

Someone who, out of a need to be active but without thinking of his or her neighbors, starts hammering nails every night between 2 and 3.

Bizarre Behavior
Someone who talks out loud to him- or herself or who screams in public.

Someone who constantly complains to the caretaker because, according to him or her, the neighbors keep moving the furniture around in his or her apartment.

Violence
Someone who attacks, apparently without motive, a helpless elderly person in public.

Someone who mistreats his or her child to the point of physical abuse.

Withdrawal
A colleague who, for days on end and apparently without reason, isolates him- or herself, refusing to speak to others even as regards questions relating to work.

Someone who locks him- or herself in, refusing to go out, keeping the curtains drawn or the shutters closed and refusing to answer the door.

References

1 Mechanic D: Some factors in identifying and defining mental illness; in J ST (ed): Mental Illness and Social Processes. New York, Harper & Row, 1967, pp 23–32.
2 Lamontagne Y: Perceptions des Québécois à l'égard de la maladie mentale. Union Méd Can 1993; 122:334–343.
3 Wolff G, Pathare S, Craig T, Leff J: Community attitudes to mental illness. Br J Psychiatry 1996; 168:183–190.
4 Hall P, Brockington IF, Levings J, Murphy C: A comparison of responses to the mentally ill in two communities. Br J Psychiatry 1993;162:99–108.
5 Eker D: Attitudes toward mental illness: Recognition, desired social distance, expected burden and negative influence on mental health among Turkish freshmen. Soc Psychiatry Psychiatr Epidemiol 1989;24:146–150.
6 Eker D, Arkar H: Experienced Turkish nurses' attitudes towards mental illness and the predictor variables of their attitudes. Int J Soc Psychiatry 1991;37:214–222.

7   Arkar H, Eker D: Influence of having a hospitalized mentally ill member in the family on attitudes toward mental patients in Turkey. Soc Psychiatry Psychiatr Epidemiol 1992;27:151–155.

8   Benkert O, Kepplinger HM, Sobota K: Psychopharmaka im Widerstreit. Berlin, Springer, 1995.

9   Angermeyer MC, Matschinger H: Lay beliefs about schizophrenic disorder: The results of a population survey in Germany. Acta Psychiatr Scand 1994;89:39–45.

10   Angermeyer MC, Däumer R, Matschinger H: Benefits and risks of psychotropic medication in the eyes of the general public: Results of a survey in the Federal Republic of Germany. Pharmacopsychiatry 1993;26:114–120.

11   Angermeyer MC, Held T, Görtler D: Pro und contra: Psychotherapie und Psychopharmakotherapie im Urteil der Bevölkerung. Psychother Psychosom Med Psychol 1993;43:286–292.

12   Moscovici S: La psychanalyse, son image et son public. Etude sur la représentation sociale de la psychanalyse. Paris, Presses Universitaires de France, 1961.

13   Herzlich C: Santé et maladie. Analyse d'une représentation sociale. Paris, Editions de l'Ecole des hautes études en sciences sociales, 1969.

14   Jodelet D: Représentation sociale: phénomènes, concept et théorie; in Moscovici S (ed): Psychologie sociale. Paris, Presses Universitaires de France, 1984, pp 357–378.

15   Goffman E: La mise en scène de la vie quotidienne. 2. Les relations en public. Paris, Editions de Minuit, 1973.

16   Cohen J, Struening EL: Opinions about mental illness in the personnel of two large mental hospitals. J Abnorm Soc Psychol 1962;64:349–360.

17   Guimon J, Ozamiz A, Viar I: Actitudes de la poblacion ante el consumo terapeutico de psicofarmacos. Actas Reunion Nacional Psiquiatr Biol 1979, pp 165–175.

Danielle Goerg, Unité d'investigation sociologique, Département de Psychiatrie, Hôpitaux Universitaires de Genève, 2, chemin du Petit-Bel-Air, CH–1225 Chêne-Bourg (Switzerland)
Tel. +41 22 305 57 51, Fax +41 22 305 57 99

Guimón J, Fischer W, Sartorius N (eds): The Image of Madness. The Public Facing Mental Illness and Psychiatric Treatment. Basel, Karger, 1999, pp 56–71

....

The General Public's Cognitive and Emotional Perception of Mental Illnesses: An Alternative to Attitude-Research

Andreas Hillert[a], *Jürgen Sandmann*[b], *Simone Christine Ehmig*[c], *Helga Weisbecker*[c], *Hans Mathias Kepplinger*[c], *Otto Benkert*[b]

[a] Medizinisch-Psychosomatische Klinik Roseneck, Prien am Chiemsee
[b] Psychiatrische Klinik der Universität Mainz and
[c] Institut für Publizistik, Johannes Gutenberg-Universität, Mainz, Germany

A recently published study by Angermeyer and Matschinger [1] showed that the rejection of mentally ill people – at least by the German public – had remained nearly unchanged for more than 20 years, notwithstanding the extensive reforms of the psychiatric system.

Social rejection of mentally ill persons by the general public is supposed not only to be an ethical problem, but to influence the psychiatric patient's perception of their disease [2, 3], their compliance and – mediated by stress resulting from stigmatization, expressed emotions and a less protective social network – their prognosis and quality of life. Therefore the attitudes of the public towards mental illness and mentally ill people have been the subject of scientific investigation for decades [4–7].

The goal of psychiatric attitude research was to evaluate the image and the extent of rejection of psychiatric patients – as shown in more or less typical vignettes – by the respondents. For this purpose questionnaires were used which derived from the Social Distance Scale the American sociologist Bogardus [8] had developed. Especially the results of surveys done by psychiatrists were interpreted to support the hypothesis of a fundamental distrust and rejection of the mentally ill by the majority of the population [9–12].

The finding that personal experience with mentally ill persons correlates with less negative attitudes has been replicated in several studies [4, 13]. Intervention studies with small and not representative samples showed the possibility of overcoming commonly held prejudice among the general public [14, 15].

It remains an open question whether this is linked with a similar development in the social behavior. But, despite some activities in this field, since the studies of Cumming and Cumming [4], Star [5] and Phillips [16] no really new and promising perspectives could be detected. According to similar results of Nunnally [7] and Kirk [17] a recent inquiry among medical students gave evidence that even persons involved in the treatment of the mentally ill maintain a distinct distance from them [18]. The results of Angermeyer and Matschinger [1] agree with those of the earlier studies [9–12]. Several questions arise: Are the results specific for the German population? What implications do these attitudes have for psychiatric patients in their daily life? What concepts of mental illness are common in the German population? Do these concepts and the negative attitudes fit? In order to answer these questions at least as regards some aspects, we present some data showing the phenomenon of mental illness as seen by the German public – at the same time as Angermeyer and Matschinger performed their studies – from a quite different point of view.

To evaluate the general public's knowledge and emotional reactions concerning mentally ill persons and psychotropic drugs, the Department of Psychiatry of the Johannes Gutenberg University Mainz had performed a representative survey in the German population [for data and discussion on psychotropic drugs, see 19, 20] and also an analysis of the popular press [21]. The questions used in the survey had been varied systematically and included cardiovascular and somatic disorders, too. Additionally, as a part of two other representative surveys, the respondents were asked to give a definition of the psychiatric terms 'schizophrenia' and 'mania'. With regard to these data we intend to give a more differentiated view of the mechanisms of awareness, perception and attitude of the phenomenon of 'mental illness' by the lay public.

Method

Representative Survey: Mental Illness and Psychotropic Drugs
In October 1992 a representative survey on the subject of 'mental illness and its treatment with psychotropic drugs' was carried out in Germany. The sampled population, 2,176 people, including females and males of German nationality who were at least 16 years old, was selected by a quota sample design, in which each interviewer was told the criteria and how many people she/he had to select. The population survey was carried out by the Institut für Demoskopie Allensbach.

The survey was conducted in the form of a personal, fully structured interview. To prevent systematic errors in collecting the data, for example that respondents cease to answer questions because of the sensitive topic, or to give consistent answers not related to their personal view, the number of questions was reduced by splitting them into two equal groups.

The questions were mixed with questions on other topics in order to ensure that the primary goal of the survey be obscure. In order to make the interview more lively different sorts of questions were used (card games, lists of items, drawings). We tried to avoid any discriminating or offending vocabulary.

Representative Survey: Psychiatric Diagnoses

In two representative multithematic surveys also carried out by the Institut für Demoskopie Allensbach and performed according to the same procedure as survey 1 in May 1992, the respondents (1,052 and 1,074) were asked to give a definition of the psychiatric terms 'schizophrenia' and 'mania'. The answers were registered and afterwards related to categories according to their medical correctness.

Results

The respondents were asked by whom they had been treated in recent years and they were shown a list of all medical specialists including psychiatrists, psychotherapists, psychologists, 'Nervenärzte' (in Germany 'Nervenärzte' are both specialized in neurology and in psychiatry). Altogether 132 of the respondents, that is 7.3%, stated that they had been treated by at least one mental-health professional (table 1).

In the course of the interview, the respondent's own experiences with somatic and mental diseases were explicated. Altogether 6% of the interviewees admitted that they had claimed professional help because of 'some sort of mental problems'. Remarkably only 33% of those who had been treated by a psychiatrist, psychotherapist, psychologist or 'Nervenarzt' (table 1) answered this question positively. Also 27 of the 47 respondents who had been treated by a psychotherapist, according to their own answers, now denied ever to have had serious psychological problems.

Table 2 shows the results of two questions: first whether the respondent had personally contact with a person suffering from a somatic or mental disease that was described in a short vignette. In the other question, a number of cards, on each of which a medical term or diagnosis was written, were presented and the respondent was asked to select the cards 'with a disease, someone, you know very well, has or had been suffering from'. With regard to the frequencies of diseases like heart attack, rheumatism or diabetes, it was not surprising that more than half of the interviewees knew at least one person suffering from it. As to the medical diagnosis and the vignettes of rheumatism and diabetes, the diagnosis and the corresponding symptomatology were equally known by the respondents. But only some of the respondents who stated that they knew someone who had suffered a 'heart attack' also said that they knew someone who had suffered a 'failure of blood supply to the

Table 1. Consultation of medical professionals (n = 2,176)

	%
Family doctor	84.4
Dentist	79.6
General practitioner	26.3
Ear, nose and throat specialist	25.1
Internist	20.5
Orthopedist	17.3
Dermatologist	16.7
Surgeon	13.0
'Nervenarzt' [1]	3.6
Psychotherapist	2.2
Psychologist	1.0
Psychiatrist	0.5

Question: 'Several medical doctors and other medical health professionals are written down on the list. Who was consulted by you during the last years?'

[1] As to the 78 people treated by a 'Nervenarzt' it remained open whether they consulted him because of a mental or a neurological problem. 17 of these had also consulted other 'psycho'-therapists; answering another question 20 declared to have psychological problems and 24 admitted to having taken psychotropic drugs. Notwithstanding some overlap, these data give evidence that at least half of this group had been treated for mental problems.

heart muscle'. Similarly the term 'depression' was used in a rather imprecise way. Only two thirds of those who mentioned they knew a depressed person, also said that they knew 'someone, who is sad, hopeless and tired of life, without any convincing reason'.

Less than 10% of the respondents knew people suffering from schizophrenia or mania. This small group was relatively well informed about diagnosis and symptomatology of these mental diseases. They also knew that schizophrenia is characterized not only by first-rank symptoms like paranoia and acoustic hallucinations, but also by withdrawal and autism (negative symptomatology). If only one third of the population knows the symptomatology of a clinical depression, less than 10% know that of schizophrenia and mania from their own personal experience. It means that the majority gets their information on mental diseases only 'second hand', for example from the media. We also asked whether the respondents could recollect articles in the press, or reports on television or on the radio on the subject of 'health problems' and somatic

Table 2. Personal contact with patients suffering from somatic and/or mental disorders: knowledge of diagnoses and symptomatologies (n = 2,176)

	%
Rheumatism	62.3
Painful disease of the joints, muscles, nerves and tendons, arthrosis: someone cannot move without pain	59.5
Diabetes	60.6
The level of blood sugar is too high: someone suffering from it has to be on a diet and possibly needs injections every day	58.6
Sudden heart attack	60.0
Sudden infarct in the heart muscle: the heart is suddenly insufficiently supplied with blood	44.9
Depression	33.8
Someone is very sad, hopeless and tired of life without a real reason	19.4
Schizophrenia	7.1
Illusion and hallucination: someone imagines to be persecuted by other people, hears voices nobody else can hear and tastes poison in food	6.5
Someone, having been very successful in the past, has cut himself off from other people in recent years, he is unable to do anything; he stays in bed the whole day	7.9
Mania	5.4
Someone is agitated, immoderately overestimates his abilities and imagines to possess many things he really does not have	9.3

Question: 'On the index cards health problems and diseases are written down. Some of them can be found quite often, others are rare. Please pick out the cards, describing something someone you know well is or was suffering from.' Initially only cards with descriptions of symptomatologies were given. After questions concerning other subjects a similar question was asked again by using the cards with the diagnoses.

and mental disorders quoted above (table 3). Reports on AIDS and alcohol dependence were recollected by more than half, high blood pressure, diabetes and dependency on tablets by half of the respondents. Schizophrenia and mania as the subject of a report could be remembered only by 10%, depression by 21%.

If the questions were modified, shifting from objective reports to emotional stories, for example 'Have you ever read in the press or heard on television or the radio that a mentally ill person has committed a violent crime?', over 60% could recollect such contributions (table 3). Articles about serious side

Table 3. Recollection of media reports on diseases: newspapers and magazines, radio and television (n = 2,176)

	%
Question 1	
AIDS	81
Alcoholism	61
High blood pressure	48
Diabetes	44
Addiction to prescribed drugs	43
Arthrosis/joint disease/'rheumatism'	41
Insomnia/sleep disturbances	37
Depression	21
Paranoia/schizophrenia	11
Someone feels persecuted by other people, hears voices nobody else can hear and tastes poison in food	11
Mania	9
Question 2	
Alcoholism, that someone has ruined his life by drinking too much	74
That a mentally ill person had committed a violent crime	64
That someone became addicted to prescribed drugs	50
About people suffering from side effects of medications	46
About a lawsuit against the pharmacological industry because of the side effects of their medication	37
About someone who has ruined his career because of an addiction to drugs	32
About mentally ill persons who became able to lead a normal life by taking their medication	17

Question 1: 'Returning to health problems and diseases: about which of the following problems have you heard or read, I mean in newspapers or magazines, on the radio or on television?' Index-cards were given.

Question 2: 'Some subjects which are regularly discussed in newspapers and magazines are on this list. About which of them have you read?'

effects of medications, especially the problem of dependence, are similarly well preserved in the public's memory.

With regard to these results it is not surprising that there is less willingness to have a conversation on the subject of mental disorders like schizophrenia or drug dependence, as is the case with AIDS, even among family members and friends (table 4). In case someone suffered from one of these problems,

Table 4. Readiness to talk about somatic and mental diseases of relatives (n = 1,088)

	With neighbors, colleagues or acquaintances %	Only with relatives or the very best friends %	Probably with nobody %	I can't say %
Hypertension/high blood pressure	64	26	7	3
Diabetes	55	36	7	3
Insomnia/sleep disturbances	51	37	10	3
Sudden heart attack	48	40	8	4
Someone, having been very successful in the past, breaks off contact with other people	22	52	20	6
Someone is very sad, hopeless and tired of life without a real reason	20	51	24	5
Someone is agitated, overestimates his abilities	19	48	27	6
Paranoia/schizophrenia	13	45	37	5
Alcoholism	11	55	31	4
Addiction to prescribed drugs	10	58	29	4
Addiction to drugs	7	52	36	4
AIDS	7	46	43	4

Question: 'In every family there might be more or less unpleasant diseases. Sometimes it might be helpful to talk to someone about it. On the other hand, certain problems should preferably remain secret. Please tell me – regarding these cards – to whom you would talk, if someone of your very close relatives suffered from one of these diseases.'

only very few people want to be involved. The respondents were asked about the therapy the different symptomatologies should receive (table 5). A strict distinction between somatic and mental diseases was obvious: while abnormal somatic conditions need the help of a doctor and some medication, nearly every person showing psychological/psychiatric symptomatology was advised to have psychotherapy. In the treatment of paranoia and hallucinations, only 8% of the population would give psychotropic drugs. In the eyes of the respondents, psychotherapy/psychoanalysis seem to be the ideal treatment for all sorts of mental problems. Respondents who had been treated because of mental problems, rated the psychopharmacological treatment significantly more positively; the preference for psychotherapy was nevertheless overwhelming.

In addition to the structured interview, in two other representative surveys adults were asked to give a definition of 'schizophrenia' and 'mania' (table 6).

Table 5. Opinions towards the treatment of health problems (n = 1,088)

	Medication %	Psycho-analysis/ psycho-therapy %	There is no treatment %	Natural remedies %	No treatment is needed, spontaneously healing %
Sudden heart attack	92	1	3	2	0
Diabetes	89	1	2	4	1
Hypertension/high blood pressure	74	1	0	21	0
Insomnia/sleep disturbances	20	15	2	49	12
Alcoholism	14	62	14	4	3
Paranoia/schizophrenia	8	77	7	2	4
Someone is very sad, hopeless and tired of life	4	65	5	8	15
Someone is agitated, overestimates his abilities immoderately	4	61	10	5	16
Someone, having been very successful in the past, breaks off contact with other people	4	68	7	6	10
AIDS	30	2	63	1	0

Question: 'Health problems can be treated in different ways, for example with medication, with natural remedies, with psychotherapy. On this paper several forms of treatment are written down. I will give you index cards with the descriptions of different health problems and diseases. Please put each card down on the treatment you consider preferable for the health problem concerned.'

Table 6. Definitions of foreign words and special terms by the lay public

	Schizophrenia (n = 1,082) %	Mania (n = 1,074) %
Correct definition	24.4	7.5
Vague definition	34.9	5.8
Incorrect definition	12.7	35.7
I don't know, no answer	28.0	51.0

In a representative survey by the Institut for Demoskopie Allensbach the respondents were asked to give definitions of 'schizophrenia' and 'mania'.

Question: 'On television and in the newspapers foreign words are frequently used. Often someone doesn't know their exact meaning. Do you know, for example, the meaning of schizophrenia/mania?'.

The answers were registered and related to categories according to their medical correctness. If the answer showed that the respondent had understood the term as something like a 'mental disease', this was considered to be correct. Only about 25% of the population had a more or less clear idea that schizophrenia means a mental disease associated with paranoia, hallucinations or 'someone has a split mind' or 'someone thinks he/she is the king of China'. Answers like 'having serious mental problems, having fears' were rated to be indifferent, 'being mad' or 'being crazy' to be wrong. That 'mania' is a distinct mental disease is nearly completely lost in the wide range of meanings associated with this term.

Discussion

According to a multicomponent conception 'attitudes are comprised not only of affect but also of cognition and connotation', to 'serve as behavioural predispositions' [22]. Since World War II, parallel to the mental-health movement, the attitude concept became highly prominent in social research. It describes mechanisms supposed to stabilize social systems, especially prejudices against fringe groups. Psychiatric attitude research hypothesized a widespread social distance, distrust to and rejection of the mentally ill by the population as a key problem for the rehabilitation of these persons [6, 23, 24].

In a recent inquiry among medical students, Rössler et al. [18] used traditional 'attitude to mentally ill' scales and discovered that the attitudes of students towards the mentally ill are as negative as the attitudes of the general public. The courses in psychiatry and contact with patients obviously did not alter the attitudes of the students. Besides the negative implications of these results a rather old question [25, 26] arises: what amount of distance to the mentally ill persons is optimal? There is very little scientific evidence, much of it contradictory, to answer this question. The results of surveys of expressed emotions and social networks partly touch this subject. Do psychiatrists and scientists engaged in the psychiatric attitude research really expect the lay public, medical students and psychiatrists [17] to be happy, if their daughter marries a mentally ill person or their children are looked after by someone who has been in psychiatric care? From a professional point of view these questions cannot be answered. The individual case has to be considered. That ideological aspects and some self-justifications have infiltrated psychiatric attitude research has now become evident. If the answers of some respondents indicated little social distance to the mentally ill, authors regularly considered whether these results might be biased by social desirability [27]. The same must be discussed concerning the psychiatric attitude research itself [9, 24].

Using 'attitude' scales and vignettes introduced by Star [5] in 1953 in order to show typical symptomatologies of mentally ill patients, more or less all surveys confirmed the hypothesis of a fundamental social distance [1, 4, 7, 12, 18, 25, 26]. The constant results are somehow astonishing in view of the fundamental changes in psychiatry since 1953: psychopharmacological treatment, a new understanding of genetic and neurophysiological processes involved in mental illnesses and a reform in psychiatric-health care systems with the reintegration of mentally ill persons being the main goal of modern psychiatry.

There have been different opinions about the reasons for this dissatisfying situation. While in the first decades of psychiatric attitude research sociological hypotheses [stigmatization and rejection of groups with nonconformist behavior, 24] were discussed, now the influence of popular media, especially women's magazines, seems to be of special interest [21, 28, 29]. According to the results of our survey the majority remembers – on television or radio – stories in conformity with this stereotype, while medical reports on mental diseases are significantly less prominent (table 3). People who are not in contact with mentally ill persons have few resources for objective information. Reports in general newspapers – discussing the subject fairly – are read only by a minority [21]. In the curriculum of German and Austrian schools the phenomenon of mental illness does not exist [30].

In psychiatry and in social sciences the question of whether negative attitudes towards the mentally ill are a fact or an artifact, caused by the methodology of attitude research, remained unanswered [11]. It has to be considered that the structure, terminology and the context of the interview influence the results [31]. Minor modifications of the formulation of the questions can cause highly significant differences, as shown in our survey: if the interviewee had to choose one of several alternative possibilities of treatments, only 8% would give a person suffering from schizophrenia psychopharmacological treatment. If he is asked whether these drugs should be given to the patient more than half of the respondents tend to do so (table 5). Without looking to the structural differences of the questions used in the interview, two different concepts of mental illness could be asserted.

Moreover, a systematic reexamination of the methodological limitations of the attitude concept itself is required. Especially Ajzen and Fishbein [22] have pointed out that 'attitudes' uttered in questionnaires – or verbal behavior – do not necessarily correlate with the behavior shown in social situations. Experimental studies established a rather low attitude-behavior relation. The different situative and psychological factors influencing the rating on the one and the social behavior on the other hand are quite difficult to evaluate. The amount of influence each of these factors may have, for example the role of the raters' opinion expected by the respondent, depends on the respondent's personality and affective state. The interactions of emotional, cognitive and situative aspects are supposed to be highly complex. Their discussion leads to the theory of reasoned action, which became an interesting theoretical model with limited practical consequences. It is not clear whether the evaluated attitudes towards mentally ill persons are of value in order to predict social behaviour to the mentally ill. Because of the huge amounts of time and manpower necessary and methodological problems, no systematic evaluations of the social distance towards mentally ill persons in real life have been carried out.

One aspect closely related to the attitudes is the cognitive perception, that is to say the illness conception of the population. Star [5] found in the early days of attitude research that only a minority could identify the patients shown in the vignettes to be mentally ill and that those who did showed a more accentuated rejection. Although in the meantime some contrasting results had been obtained [24], the findings of Star were replicated several times [13]. The implications of these findings for the attitude conception were neglected notwithstanding the fact that in discussions this seems to be important.

Lay person's assumptions about mental illness were investigated independently from the attitude research, too. In western societies fantasies of magical and moral causes of mental illness are quite vivid [2]. In one study [32] lay persons and patients in psychiatric hospitals in Germany and in the United States were asked directly: while Germans tended to view the phenomenon as inherited, enduring, difficult to cure, and not influenced by personal effort, the Americans tended to see the problem to be caused by difficult circumstances, relatively curable and likely to improve by means of therapeutic efforts. Accordingly, the German patients tended to deny being mentally ill significantly more often. Of course in this study several methodological problems have to be discussed, too: different populations, different groups of patients and a different understanding or semantic connotation of the terms used in the inquiry.

In this context, the results of our survey [similar to 33] represent a conception of mental illness that differs both from the professional point of view but also from the hypothesis of attitude research. Different aspects in our study can be distinguished: (1) knowledge, (2) personal experience with mental illness and (3) illness concepts including ideas of prognosis and treatment.

(1) Public knowledge: About 25% of the respondents were able to give a correct explanation of 'schizophrenia', only 10% could explain the term 'mania' as some sort of mental illness (table 6). The ignorance of psychiatric diagnoses by the majority cannot not be interpreted in the sense that the respondents have no experience with the phenomenon of mental illness. Regarding the term of 'mental illness' Stumme [34, 35] could show in a semantic analysis that the lay public uses different words in colloquial speech to distinguish several degrees of illness severity. But the conclusion of Stumme that the lay public is able to

distinguish 'deviating mental behaviour in a very differentiated way' seems to be premature: to distinguish different forms of deviating behavior does not necessarily mean that they are recognized to be caused by a mental illness.

(2) Personal experience: Less than 10% of the respondents admitted to having experience with serious psychological problems. The members of this small group could hardly define whether they had been treated by a psychiatrist, psychologist or psychotherapist because of a 'real' mental illness. The problem of stigmatization of mentally ill persons and corresponding cautious behavior [2] may have influenced these results.

(3) Illness concepts implicate the form of treatment. Psychotherapy is supposed by the majority of our respondents to be adequate to all mental disorders shown in the vignettes, even to a paranoid schizophrenia. It seems to be a rather sympathetic 'attitude': not psychotropic drugs thought to calm down the patients without a real therapeutic effect [19, 20], but a conversation and support by a psychotherapist will help. There is less evidence that the patients portrayed in the vignettes were identified as sick persons suffering from a medical disorder according to the psychiatric systems. Something like a concept of 'mental illness' can be detected only in a very rudimentary way. While a psychiatrist makes the diagnosis 'schizophrenia', the lay public sees a poor, sad man/woman, having serious problems and 'stress'.

When attitudes and the concepts of mental disorders are compared with each other, it becomes evident that there is not much medical knowledge available on these subjects and that the concepts are without an elaborate theory and quite vague, determined by a rather naive view of the patient as someone who has real problems, is sad and needs help. If only a minority knows the symptomatologies of mental illnesses and meets the requirement of recognition of a mentally ill, what implications do the attitudes of the majority have?

Especially the schema concepts open new perspectives for a more differentiated view and understanding of the interaction of emotional and cognitive aspects subsumed in the attitude concept. Schema concepts are developed by empirical psychology in order to describe the basic mechanisms of the brain functioning both regarding cognitions and emotions [for an overview and discussion, see 36–38]. The definition by Crocker et al. [37] catches the main aspects: 'A schema is an abstract or generic knowledge structure stored in memory that specifies the defining features and relevant attributes of some stimulus domains and the interrelation among the structures.' A cognitive or affective schema is identified and activated by specific stimuli. Affective schemata can be activated directly or via a corresponding cognitive perception [39, 40]. In contrast to the attitude theories, the schema concepts make it possible to look separately at cognitive and affective aspects of behavior. Regarding the different aspects of knowledge, perception and emotions concerning 'mental illness' different cognitive and affective schemata can be supposed.

Cognitive Schemata

C 1: 'a person needs help'. Somebody has problems, feels unhappy, needs help and support. This schema determines the responding behavior in our study: as long as a subject sees a psychopathological symptomatology caused by a process familiar to his own experience – or maintains a psychological illness concept (having stress, being sad because of something) – C 1 will be activated. Intraindividual differences in being introspective and reflecting psychological phenomena also determine the thresholds between C 1 and C 2.

C 2: 'a mentally ill person'. Quite different to C 1 'a person needs help', the stimuli activating the schema of 'a mentally ill person' include the coincidence of behavioral aspects like aggressiveness, dangerousness, being out of control, no real communication is possible, the behavior of a person is incomprehensible and incalculable.

Beside, and as to some aspects independently, from cognitive schemata, the emotional reaction towards the phenomenon of mental illness is determined by specific affective reactions or schemata [39, 40].

Affective Schemata

A 1: 'I like this person'. The emotional reaction towards a person who needs help regularly contains emotional warmth, hospitality and the feeling of 'I like this person'. Of course other aspects, body size, expression on her/his face, clothing and behavior (directly asking for help, being reserved) and the situation (being with this person in a forest far away from any other people, seeing this person being treated against her/his will with psychotropic drugs by psychiatrists) have an influence on the emotional perception.

A 2: 'the person is not good and may be/is dangerous'. If aspects of the person or her/his behavior indicate dangerousness, the feeling of 'not good' and the very strong emotional schema of fear (and reaction) will be activated. The studies of Cumming and Cumming [4], Phillips [16] and of others have shown that the severity of deviant behavior, agitation and aggression and any hint that a person has been in psychiatric treatment indicate dangerousness at least in the eyes of the respondents [25] and determine negative 'attitudes' and rejection.

Meeting a 'mentally ill person' (for example a person suffering from schizophrenia, DSM-IV 295.30) will activate different cognitive and affective schemata, which are in hierarchic interaction. If an attractive young schizophrenic girl talks about being pursued by a psychiatrist the cognitive and affective schemata (A 1/C 1) will correspond. An unkempt strong man, showing the same symptomatology, may cause some schemata ambivalence: seen at a safe distance (for example in a vignette) he may be perceived as A 1/C 1, too; meeting him alone in the street, a spontaneously activated affective reaction A 2 will determine a cognitive perception according to C 2.

'If there is indeed a separation between affect and cognition, then it is not surprising, that ... attitudes research ... has not been terribly successful.' This statement by Zajonc [39], focusing on the interaction of cognitive and affective schemata, also seems to be the key for understanding the stagnation of psychiatric attitude research. The contradicting results in this field, the discrepancies between 'negative attitudes' towards mentally ill persons [1] and the sensitive and introspective illness conceptions, as shown in our survey, can easily be explained by the simple fact that there is no specific or single attitude to the phenomenon of mental illness or the 'mentally ill' held by the lay public. The reasons are that firstly mental illness is not recognized as a distinct phenomenon (as seen by mental health professionals and diagnostic systems like DSM-IV). Secondly, the strong affective aspects of any 'attitude', which are determined only partly by the psychopathology but also by a wide spectrum of other personal aspects of the patient, gender, the situative context and many more, are neglected.

The dynamic nature of schemata may also open up new perspectives: a schema is not a static and irreversible construct. Motivating the subject to re-activate the contents of the actual schema, it is steadily modified by assimilation and accommodation [41]. An example fitting into our context is the training of medical students and psychiatrists. This training goes along with a substantial development of cognitive schemata: the A 1 schema will be 'professionalized', enriched with diagnostic entities of current psychiatric classification systems. The white coat, the professional distance of a doctor and the training of strategies to handle persons with deviating behavior are due to different and new thresholds also of the C 2 schemata (there are less 'unexplained' symptomatologies) and with this the affective schemata A 2 [21, 42]. Nevertheless, the 'negative' affective schemata A 2 will be pushed back but not loosened. Also psychiatrists (at least the authors) have some fears and negative emotions when confronted with a strong and aggressive schizophrenic patient. That attitudes of medical students and professionals [17, 18, 43] are not significantly 'better' than those of the lay public can easily be explained by this phenomenon: when A 2 is activated (the own child is to be looked after by a mentally ill person) the 'professionalized' cognitive schema C 1, because of the hierarchic structure, is switched off or at least dominated by a strong negative emotional quality.

A 2 is the limiting factor of any approach in order to improve knowledge and 'attitudes' towards the phenomenon of mental illness. If active, the subject will have no resources for an adequate cognitive perception of new information. On the other hand, according to the motivational component of schemata, a fundamental interest in understanding the mechanisms causing emotional problems and possibilities of treating psychopathological symptoms can be expected (C 1).

Conclusion

Whether the public attitudes towards the mentally ill are good or bad and whether they have changed in the last decades or not cannot be answered because of the methodological problems discussed in this paper. The concepts and methods of 'traditional' attitude research are unsuited for any further progress in this field, because they do not sufficiently discriminate aspects of emotional and cognitive perception. The schema concepts open a new understanding of the perception of the phenomenon of mental illness and therefore of further studies and educational programs in this field, too.

References

1   Angermeyer MC, Matschinger D: Social distance towards the mentally ill: Results of representative surveys in the Federal Republic of Germany. Psychol Med 1997;27:131–141.
2   Johnson S, Orrell M: Insight and psychosis: A social perspective. Psychol Med 1995;25:515–520.
3   Kemp R, David A: Psychosis: Insight and compliance. Curr Opin Psychiatry 1995;8:357–361.
4   Cumming E, Cumming J: Closed Ranks: An Experiment in Mental Health. Cambridge, Harvard University Press, 1957.
5   Star SA: The Public's Idea about Mental Illness. Chicago, National Opinion Research Center, 1955.
6   Hollingshead AB, Redlich FC: Social Class and Mental Illness. New York, Wiley, 1958.
7   Nunnally JC: Popular Conceptions of Mental Health. New York, Holt, Rinehart & Winston, 1961.
8   Bogardus ES: A social distance scale. Sociol Soc Res 1933;17:265–271.
9   Brockmann J, D'Arcy C, Edmonds L: Facts or artifacts? Changing public attitudes toward the mentally ill. Soc Sci Med 1979;13A:673–682.
10 Bissland JH: The Torledo study of attitudes toward mental illness: A Q-methodological approach; in Burgon M (ed): Communication Yearbook 5. An Annual Review Published by the International Communication Association. New Brunswick, Transaction Books, 1982, pp 783–806.
11 McPherson JG, Cocks FJ: Attitudes toward mental illness: Influence of data collection procedures. Soc Psychiatry 1983;18:57–60.
12 Brockington IF, Hall P, Levings J, Murphy Ch: The community's tolerance of the mentally ill. Br J Psychiatry 1993;162:93–99.
13 Ingamells S, Goodwin AM, John C: The influence of psychiatric hospital and community residence labels on social rejection of the mentally ill. Br J Clin Psychol 1996;35:359–367.
14 Link BG, Cullen FF, Frank J: Social rejection of former mental patients: Understanding why labels matter. Am J Sociol 1987;92:1461–1500.
15 Voges B, Rössler W: Beeinflusst die gemeindenahe psychiatrische Versorgung das Bild vom psychisch Kranken in der Gesellschaft? Neuropsychiatrie 1995;9:144–151.
16 Phillips DL: Identification of mental illness: Its consequences for rejection. Community Ment Health J 1967;3:262–266.
17 Kirk S: The impact of labelling on rejection of the mentally ill. An experimental study. J Health Soc Behav 1974;15:108–117.

18   Rössler W, Salize HJ, Trunk V, Voges B: Die Einstellung von Medizinstudenten gegenüber psychisch Kranken. Nervenarzt 1996;67:757–764.
19   Benkert O, Kepplinger HM, Sobota K, Ehmig SC, Hillert A, Sandmann J, Weissbecker H: Psychopharmaka im Widerstreit. Berlin, Springer, 1995.
20   Benkert O, Graf-Morgenstern M, Hillert A, Sandmann J, Ehmig SC, Weissbecker H, Kepplinger HM, Sobota K: Public opinions on psychotropic drugs: An analysis of the factors influencing acceptance or rejection. J Nerv Ment Dis 1997;85:152–158.
21   Hillert A, Sandmann J, Ehmig SC, Sobota K, Weisbecker H, Kepplinger HM, Benkert O: Psychopharmacological drugs as represented in the press: Results of a systematic analysis of newspapers and popular magazines. Pharmacopsychiatry 1996;29:67–71.
22   Ajzen I, Fishbein M: Understanding Attitudes and Predicting Social Behaviour. Englewood Cliffs, Prentice-Hall, 1980.
23   Goffmann E: Stigma. Notes on the Management of Spoiled Identity. Engelwood Cliffs, Prentice-Hall, 1963.
24   Crocetti GM, Spiro HR, Siassi I: Contemporary attitudes toward mental illness. Pittsburgh, University of Pittsburgh Press, 1974.
25   Rabkin J: Public attitudes toward mental illness: A review of the literature. Schizophr Bull 1974;10:9–33.
26   Bhugra D: Attitudes towards mental illness: A review of the literature. Acta Psychiatr Scand 1989;80:1–12.
27   Wolf G, Pathare S, Craig T, Leff J: Community attitudes to mental illness. Br J Psychiatry 1996;168:183–190.
28   Schneider U, Wieser S: Der psychisch Kranke in den Massenmedien. Ergebnisse einer systematischen Inhaltsanalyse. Fortschr Neurol Psychiatr 1972;40:136–163.
29   Angermeyer MC, Siara CS: Auswirkungen der Attentate auf Lafontaine und Schäuble auf die Einstellung der Bevölkerung zu psychisch Kranken. Nervenarzt 1994;65:49–56.
30   Amann G, Baumann U: Differentielle Wissensbestände über psychische Krankheiten in den österreichischen Psychologie-Schulbüchern. Z Gesundheitspsychol 1994;2:1–24.
31   Noelle-Neumann E: Öffentliche Meinung. Die Entdeckung der Schweigespirale. 3. Frankfurt a. M., Ullstein, 1991.
32   Townsend JM: Cultural Conception and Mental Illness. Chicago, University of Chicago Press, 1978.
33   Angermeyer MC, Däumer R, Matschinger H: Benefits and risks of psychotropic medication in the eyes of the general public: Results of a survey in the Federal Republic of Germany. Pharmacopsychiatry 1993;26:114–120.
34   Stumme W: Was heisst 'Geisteskrankheit'? Nervenarzt 1970;41:294–298.
35   Stumme W: Die differenzierten Vorstellungen des Laien zum Problemkreis psychischer Erkrankungen. Eine Kritik der Vorurteilsforschung; Dissertation, Cologne, 1972.
36   Fiske ST, Linville PW: What does the schema concept by us? Pers Soc Psychol Bull 1980;6:543–557.
37   Crocker J, Fiske ST, Taylor SE: Schematic base of belief change; in Eiser JR (ed): Attitudinal Judgement. Berlin, Springer, 1984, pp 197–226.
38   Sachse R: Zielorientierte Gesprächspsychotherapie. Göttingen, Hogrefe, 1992.
39   Zajonc RB: Feeling and thinking. Preferences need no inferences. Am Psychol 1980;35:151–175.
40   Zajonc RB: On the primacy of affect. Am Psychol 1984;39:117–123.
41   Piaget J: Die Äquilibration der kognitiven Strukturen. Stuttgart, Klett, 1976.
42   Sandmann J, Hillert A, Benkert O: The public opinion on the therapeutic value of psychotropic versus cardiac drugs. Pharmacopsychiatry 1993;26:194.
43   Hillert A, Sandmann J, Angermeyer MC, Däumer R: Die Einstellung von Medizinstudenten zur Behandlung mit Psychopharmaka. Der Wandel der Einstellung im Verlauf des Studiums. Psychiatr Prax 1994;21:64–69.

Dr. Dr. Andreas Hillert, Medizinisch-Psychosomatische Klinik Roseneck,
Center for Behavioral Medicine, Am Roseneck 6, D-83209 Prien am Chiemsee (Germany)
Tel. +49 8051 680, Fax +49 8051 683690

Guimón J, Fischer W, Sartorius N (eds): The Image of Madness. The Public Facing Mental
Illness and Psychiatric Treatment. Basel, Karger, 1999, pp 72–84

....

'Cooperating', 'Fighting against' or 'Letting Go' in the Therapeutic Context: Social Logic of Parents with Psychologically Disturbed Children

Marie-Noëlle Schurmans[a], *Nicolas Duruz*[b, c]

[a] Faculty of Psychology and Sciences of Education, University of Geneva,
[b] University of Fribourg, and
[c] University of Lausanne, Switzerland

Two strong premises underlie the different contributions to the topic of
public opinion on mental illness: on one hand, the negative public attitudes
towards 'mental illness' as well as regarding psychiatrists and their various
treatments, on the other hand, the idea of an underlying distance between
the professional knowledge of psychiatrists and common sense knowledge of
mental illness.

We will tackle this wide-ranging issue from a specific angle: the therapeutic
relationship. Indeed, we think that this relationship is all too often construed
as being the encounter between legitimate knowledge – i.e. the therapist's –
and an absence of, or at the best, limited knowledge attributed to the patient.
The medical field, in complete awareness of the importance of the therapeutic
relationship, has often emphasized the necessity to give public access to medical
theories and treatments. Of course, the unfamiliar and mysterious aspects of
medical activities often induce suspicion or even sometimes antagonism to
medical staff. Cramer [1] describes this effect in the following terms: 'For the
medical staff the most obvious of these harmful incidences is the fact that
patients increasingly refuse to undergo our treatments. We often come across
rejection of prescribed treatments that become public health problems.'
According to Cramer, one of the causes of the rejection lies in a lack of
information given by the therapist to the patient regarding the illness and the

purpose of the treatment. We propose a complementary approach based on recognizing the patient's personal knowledge and the necessity that the therapist should take it into consideration.

Material and Methods

The research we refer to [2][1] stems from an issue developed during clinical interventions in the course of children's psychiatric treatment. To be more precise the research focuses on analyzing social representations of children's mental illness as seen by parents who are personally involved in the arduous process of dealing with their children's inappropriate behavior, medical diagnosis and therapeutic treatments.

These are parents of children who attended, for at least 1 year, the Psychotherapeutic Day Center of the Children's Hospital in Lausanne. This center aims to keep the children in their family and social environment by providing an intermediate stage between day care and full-time hospitalization. It cares for children with severe personality problems, mainly of psychotic or prepsychotic origin. Eighty-four cases met the criteria developed in our research, but only 32 were analyzed as a result of parents refusing, moving away or not replying to our appeal. Our research material comprises transcriptions of semidirected interviews (unlimited in time) with both parents[2] based on their life story. The idea was to reconstruct the memory of situations in which handling emotions – in an extremely emotional context – as well as building up knowledge and know-how are prominent.

Our hypotheses were drawn up at different levels. First of all we wanted to study the contents of parents' representations from the point of view of their genesis, their development and their organization. We then dug into the parents' valorizations not only regarding the sources of their information but also the explanatory models they were given in order to shed light on the degree of compatibility between their representations of the etiology and the principal theoretical guidelines accepted by therapists. Finally, we focused our approach on the link between the contents of representations, the valorizations and the actions taken: relationships established by parents with the various therapeutic processes offered for the benefit of their children were therefore studied.

Because of the limited space we have at our disposal we cannot describe all the dimensions of this particular research and the independent variables we used for analyzing data, nor can we define the analysis technique: we will refer to them only as regards the observations selected for the remainder of this article. We have decided to emphasize certain results directly connected with issues shared by various authors. We will therefore focus on the question of parents' negative attitudes towards therapists and then move on to the problem of compatibility between parents' representations and the dominant models therapists retain. Finally, we examine the link between parents' valorizations and representations and the social grounding of their organization.

[1] This research (request No. 1114-40810.94) was made possible thanks to fundings from the Fonds National de la Recherche Scientifique Suisse.
[2] Our initial idea of interviewing both parents was not possible if the parents were divorced or if one of the parents was not available.

Results

Attitudes towards Professionals

What type of professionals did the parents meet throughout the treatment of their child and how did they assess them? Do they agree with the information, the explanations and the proposals of treatment these professionals offer or, on the contrary, do they contest them, criticize them? The degree of parental agreement with the specialist's discourse and manners comprises one of the main dimensions of our research and is based on five subthemes: skills parents assigned to professionals, trust, acknowledged efficiency, understanding information, and the amount of agreement parents share with specialists.

Our data analyses show, first of all, that the parents' positions regarding general agreement appear as a whole: assessments of 'skills', 'trust', 'efficiency', 'understanding' and 'agreement' are either totally accepted or denied. This first observation led us to construct two ideal-type variables with which global intensity of the agreement about what professionals say or do is measured: (1) for the field of special education including educators, teachers and speech therapists and (2) for the field of mental health including clinicians such as psychologists, psychotherapists, educational psychologists and psychiatrists.

The analysis of the data indicates that the parents' positions are radicalized: the agreement previously strongly accepted or totally denied is slightly inflected. This second finding encouraged us to recode our variables: strong/intermediate/low or absent agreement. Very few interviewees are located in the intermediate category with regard to clinicians or special education teachers: 3 families out of 32 are concerned. Total or strong agreement predominates for both fields. However, it is slightly more obvious as regards special education: 20 families assign it to clinicians and 24 to teachers. As for the extremely negative assessments, the ratio is the opposite since 9 families assign them to clinicians and only 5 families assign them to teachers.

Do parents agree with one field or another? We discard a positive answer insofar as a low level of agreement assigned to one field is linked to a low level of agreement in the other (χ^2 test significant at 0.01) and the same can be observed with high levels of agreement (with the same significance).

Finally, we denote that these widespread judgments are given about general categories rather than about individuals. Remarks of the interviewees apply to the legitimacy of their intervention. If most parents are convinced that these professionals are necessary, some seem to declare so without much conviction insofar that interventions of a psychotherapeutic nature seem to be automatically offered via an official system that does not allow any alternative. As for totally negative opinions, they contest the appropriateness of clinicians' interventions. This position is obviously linked to a negative representation of mental health professionals, added to a questioning of their theoretical and practical approaches, whose very intervention sometimes induces social marginalization.

These data, coming from directed parts of the interviews held with the parents, are confirmed by parts that were less directed. Here, we learn that, when parents mention meeting particular people in the mental health field, they often make sharp distinctions: 'he was particularly good, he was really incompetent'. We therefore denote that positive and negative assessments are more clearly split up: the ratio is almost the same (36 positive encounters for 34 negative ones for all interactions described by our interviewees).

Contents of these assessments are mainly related to the quality of the relationship. The leading themes of criticism apply to the 'setting' and the type of communication established by mental health professionals: there is no proper dialogue, no symmetry in the communication; they ask personal or intrusive questions that shake up the parents; communication is often focused on the present and past life of the parents and not enough on the child. Moreover, many parents feel that they are not understood or listened to properly by the clinician when discussing their worries and evaluating the child's problem. They have difficulties in assessing the professional's abilities and efficiency – they often say that they do not know what is going on – and they complain about a lack of information: explanations given are frequently too theoretical and inaccessible. One third of the parents complained that they were not helped with personal support and others that the process made them feel guilty. Finally, some clinicians are directly criticized: almost 1 family out of 4 describe the professional's attitudes as evasive and frightening. All remarks outlining individuals – be they positive or negative – are concerned with the content and the mode of communication.

What happens when parents detail their assessment on special education teachers? On the whole, the valorizations are positive for professionals met at the center: relationships are appreciated as well as the relationship established between the child, the educators and the special education teachers. Assessments were less positive for other specialized institutions they came across in the course of the child's treatment: a third of the assessments were negative and related to problems of social and professional integration of the child now or in the future.

The data on information and proposals of treatment are completed by an approach dealing with: (1) parents' social cognitive positions, in other words how their discourse relates to their knowledge (i.e. 'ignoring', 'not wanting to know', 'understanding', 'asserting', 'questioning'), (2) parents' social affective position, in other words the amount of change to the course of their life in relation to their child's problem (i.e. 'suffering', 'being angry', 'fixing limits', 'being helpless', 'being anxious', 'fighting against')[3], and (3) parents' relation to action, in other words how they took up a position, more or less 'actively', towards the dynamics of the child's treatment ('having to take actions', 'being involved', 'cooperating', 'acting against', 'taking the initiative of an action')[4].

These three dimensions were analyzed, first separately and then in pairs, with a correspondence analysis[5]. It is this last analysis that we will now comment upon.

The first factor (F1 = 32.7% of variance explained) clearly reveals an opposition concerning representations of oneself, either 'as an actor' or 'as liable to action' (becoming an agent). In all logic the second term discloses social affective positions stating 'descriptions of leading difficult life', in other words exposing various problems without reacting to them. From the point of view of social cognitive positions, the problem of denying professional abilities appears as well as asserting parallel knowledge clearly separate from the specialist's knowledge. However, representations of oneself as an actor, both initiating and being responsible for actions, from the point of view of social affective positions, pairs with outlining feelings connected with various reactions involving either rebellious feelings or personal therapy; from the point of view of social cognitive positions, we frequently denote statements on a lack of personal knowledge.

The second factor (F2 = 17.2% of variance explained) mainly deals with the way in which the interviewees assess their relationships with other partners of action, chiefly clinicians and special education teachers. We observe, on one hand, a clear attitude of opposition: as a reaction, opposition does not imply parents' involvement in action; on other occasions, despite being conflicting, opposition does not exclude cooperation. On the other hand, we denote a set of imprecise and at times varying attitudes, where an absence of cooperation with the therapists predominates as well as an absence of initiative and the feeling of being manipulated.

The two factors explain 50% of the variance and provide the means to interpret three different types of logic: (1) An *acting logic* implying the feeling that something has to be done, that some form of initiative should be taken, but at the same time indicating incomplete knowledge and analyzing the situation in terms of problems, all this arising either from rebellion or opposition, or in the

---

[3] The components of these two dimensions were revealed through a correspondence analysis established by SPAD-T (Système portable d'analyse de données textuelles – Portable System for Analyzing Textual Data) [see 3].

[4] These categories are the indicators of this last dimension: they are located by a thematic content analysis.

[5] We undertook our analyses using the TRI–2 program [see 4, 5].

course of a personal change or therapy. An *agent logic* that can be divided as follows: (2) an *agent logic of the victim* = the feeling of being liable to action paired with a reactionless statement on the difficult life being led; in this case professionals are not rejected, but parents credit them with the initiative of actions they do not feel responsible for, and (3) an *agent logic of retreat* = the existence of an other kind of knowledge is emphasized, parallel to scientific knowledge which is therefore questioned; in this case the idea of cooperation (joint action) is not taken into consideration – professionals are considered 'out of bounds'.

Compatibility between Lay Knowledge and Professional Knowledge

What kind of knowledge do parents refer to, during our interviews, after years of meetings and counselling by specialists of therapeutic and educational treatment of their children? Instead of considering the notion of a 'distance' between their knowledge and specialists' knowledge, we put forth the question of their compatibility or their antagonism. We do not think that it is a question of distance or closeness between therapist and public knowledge. On the contrary, we think the issue concerns mutual acceptance of knowledge acquired by different protagonists involved in the therapeutic relationship. We tackled this issue by investigating parents' representations of the etiology of their child's disorder, on one hand, and of the therapeutic treatments considered appropriate for their child, on the other hand, and whether or not these treatments were actually offered.

As for etiology, we classified the parents' conceptions using four axes composed of two opposite components [6].

(1) The 'ontological/relational' axe distinguishes between an ontological pole, on one hand, frequently referring to physical aspects, focusing on the existence of the illness and implying understanding in terms of injury combined with a qualitative option (the illness turns the person into something else) and a relational pole, on the other hand, focusing on the person who is ill, implying understanding in terms of functioning combined with a quantitative analysis of disruption between mankind and his environment (illness makes the person different).

(2) The 'exogenous/endogenous' axe opposes a conception of illness where the causes are associated with something foreign interfering (either natural or cultural) with a conception of illness where the causes (somatic or psychological) are in the person.

(3) The 'additive/subtractive' axe distinguishes illness seen as a supplementary element (something extra) and illness conceived as something missing (negative, absence of, lack of).

(4) The 'evil/beneficial' axe, finally, demarcates a conception of illness considered as something harmful, hurtful, noxious, missing, and a conception

of illness entailing an ambivalent or positive meaning (illness must retain some meaning as it is seen, in some cases, as an event that can intensify or contribute to gaining a wealth of experience).

For the therapeutic models we followed the logical distinctions proposed by the same author.

(1) In the 'allopathic/homeopathic' axe, the 'allopathic' pole refers to treatments that aim at stifling symptoms with their opposites, the purpose being to destroy the pathogenic agent without destroying the illness. As for the 'homeopathic' pole, it refers to treatments that seek to reactivate the symptoms using elements of the same kind, the purpose here being to encourage actions alleviating the organism's defense mechanisms. We would like to underline the fact that, as far as psychological disorders are concerned, and in particular with children, we had to extend Laplantine's definitions. Terms like 'homeopathic' and 'allopathic' are therefore used in a figurative sense and do not refer, or only occasionally, to these forms of medicine in a literal sense.

(2) The 'additive/subtractive' axe distinguishes treatments that try to give back what the illness has taken away from treatments that try to eliminate what illness has brought on.

(3) The 'exorcist/endorcist' axe demarcates a representation of the therapist as a combatant fighting against the illness, and a representation that sees him as an assistant supporting the patient throughout his relationship with his illness.

(4) Last of all, the 'sedative/excitable' axe opposes treatments that sedate, inhibits with treatments that stimulate, excite.

Our data suggest that the 'ontological/relational' and the 'exogenous/endogenous' axes are clearly discriminant for etiology. The 'additive/subtractive' axe also presents a clear systematization of opposite positions, but the multivariable analyses that we undertook do not grant enough evidence to ascertain a distribution of additive and subtractive conceptions that equates the two previous axes. As for treatments, parents' conceptions differ clearly on two axes: 'allopathic/homeopathic' and 'sedative/excitable'. But, yet again, the multivariable analyses only emphasize a correlation with conceptions on the etiology for the first pair of opposites.

Correspondence analyses were completed in several phases; the last phase that only takes into consideration the most discriminant variables accounts for an explanation with a percentage of 63.4 for F1 and 15.3 for F2. The results reveal a definite opposition between the two main models that our hypotheses forecasted.

Regarding conceptions on the causes of the child's disorder, we denote an opposition between a 'substantialistic' logic and a 'functional' logic. The first logic is based on an ontological model: causes of disorder, essentially physical causes conceived in terms of 'being', are located in the person. The second logic is based on a relational model: causes conceived in terms of loss of equilibrium, are connected to an 'accident' owing to something foreign interfering. Therapeutic orientations, valorized or depreciated by parents, produce the following opposition: on one hand, we find methods that aim at taking actions against the symptoms and at eradicating the 'evil', methods that are linked, in our data, with a substantialistic logic regarding etiology; on the other hand, we observe methods connected to a functional logic regarding etiology that try to help 'nature' find its equilibrium, by understanding symptoms and not suppressing diversity but by enhancing its positive aspects.

Moreover, we are able to display correspondences between these forms of organization of representations and the two principal schemata of intelligibility that organize knowledge and, for historical reasons, have always been edge to edge in specialized fields: a biomedical conception and a social psychological conception of illness.

According to the first conception, the causes of pathologies are conceived in ontological terms, fitting in with the basis of our contemporary western medicine: body and mind are separate, the latter referring to metaphysics and the former to physics. This option matches approaches of illness based on essence, propelled by the idea of establishing a classification of illnesses, approaches based on anatomy and pathology, aiming at 'locating' pathologies, and approaches regarding various etiologies based on identifying the specific cause of each symptom. We would like to underline the fact that this conception does not emphasize either the exogenous or the endogenous causes of disorders: the causes of illness are harmful, natural agents that are either connected to mankind's relationship with physical, chemical or biochemical environment, in the first case, or with assumptions on nature, predispositions, genotype, innate or acquired potential, in the second case. However, the ontological etiology, as seen in our data, refers mostly to the endogenous aspects of the causes of illness. Last of all, the classical medical model chiefly places most emphasis on allopathic treatment which corresponds to 'aggressive assault therapies' aiming at the extermination of illness – as described by Laplantine [6].

The second conception of illness – the social psychological conception – is mainly sustained by theories developed in specific fields such as psychoanalysis, systemic therapy or antipsychiatry. This option equates other medical trends that appear throughout the history of medical thought: the idea is to pursue the causes of illness more in terms of the efforts the organism produces in order to fight back than in terms of the intrusion of a pathological agent, to conceive illness more in terms of excess and lack of something than in terms of being someone else, to be aware of the organizational processes and the functional disorganization of the person in his setting. Such social psychological approaches, particularly predominant in the field of mental pathologies, tend to adopt a conception referring to the exogenous aspects of disorders that can be conceived both as natural and cultural; however, some psychoanalytical theories, and mostly systemic analysis models, have also welcomed approaches of disorders in terms of social genesis.

In the field of social psychology, studies on representations of illness and health [7–12] have pointed to the fact that according to the initial option, apprehending illness in individual or social terms, a dual logic is generated which tends to radicalize specialized approaches; when focusing on the person who is ill, conceptions of causes are internally based on nature combined with an allopathic therapeutic option; when focusing on the social group, conceptions of causes are externally based on culture combined with a therapeutic option striving to seek out the meanings associated with symptoms.

Our data, therefore, seem to be in keeping with this double partition. Referring to the biomedical model when accounting for some of the correlations drawn from our data, we do detect almost all the predominant trends described above, and the same applies to what we have called the 'social psychological model'. But we must emphasize that at the same time people's conceptions can radically differ from scientific statements. Hence, the exogenous option, defining the causes of disorder, can be outlined in naturalistic terms, iatrogenesis, for instance, as well as in supernatural terms, evil influence, for instance. We therefore add that correspondences or differences between the main features of explanations given by people and features of explanations given to them by specialists must not be conceived according to the degree of agreement or nonagreement between conceptions, but rather according to structural compatibility or incompatibility. Consequently a social psychological discourse, for instance, elaborated by specialists in front of parents who retain a definite ontological, endogenous and allopathic option immediately appears as a confrontation or, worse still, a dialogue between the deaf.

Questioning the Therapeutic Relationship
The analysis of the following dimensions is already very enlightening: parents' levels of agreement, their relation to action, their social cognitive and social affective positions, and the main structural aspects that drive their etiologic and therapeutic representations. However, our approach aims at going beyond a simple and straightforward description of the various oppositions contrived. Indeed, our intention is not only to connect all dimensions of analyses investigated but also to bring forth explanatory propositions regarding differences observed with our interviewees.

We therefore did joint analyses of several dimensions: the degree of agreement with clinicians and special education teachers, parents' relations to action (the feeling that some form of action has to be taken; having to initiate action; having to 'fight against' someone; being acted; having to develop actions by cooperating with specialists), social cognitive and social affective positions (here we made up four discrete variables using the subjects coordinates for the first two factors yielded by analyzing our textual data and by taking into consideration their relative and absolute contributions), variables retained by analyzing representations of etiology and therapeutics (for etiology: ontological, relational, endogenous, exogenous; for therapeutics: allopathic, homeopathic), parents' plans for their child, and, last of all, prognostic for the future and assessment of the child's present condition as seen by the parents. The correspondence analysis comprises 20 active variables to which we added 3 independent nonactive variables: the child's age at the time disorders appeared, people involved in investigating the set of symptoms, and the social conditions of the family.

The interpretation of the two factors (F1 and F2 = 39.3%) is obvious since the first factor separates, on one hand, parents who admit and declare their lack of knowledge and, on the other hand, parents who testify either a 'no relation' to knowledge or knowledge that is parallel and incompatible with specialized knowledge. It is also quite obvious that we have come across an important gap concerning acceptance versus refusal or inability in establishing a proper interaction with various professionals in respect to understanding the child's disorder, its causes and ways to treat it. This points to the conditions in which parents and specialists meet and we delineate three kinds of logic:

(1) Accepting to deal with the situation, combined with acknowledging specialized knowledge, sometimes promotes relationships that look like *active opposition*. Agreement is minimal, assessment of the child's institutional record is negative, prognostic is plainly negative, and aspects that seem compatible with the classical medical model predominate (ontological etiology and refusing homeopathic-based treatments). At the heart of this opposition, two kinds of feeling of personal rebellion arise: it either pairs with personal therapy, the impression that some sort of action has to be taken, or it couples with seizing up and reactions against the specialists.

(2) On other occasions, the encounter can be based on *cooperative action* (feeling that some form of action and initiative has to be taken but also that it is necessary to cooperate with the various specialists) coupled with rebellious feelings (items such as not being understood, being angry, fighting against); here agreement with mental health professionals is strong and etiologic and therapeutic terms are compatible with the social psychological model: plans for the child include both social integration and well being. This pattern pairs with a 'privileged social condition'.

(3) In return, refusal (presence of a parallel knowledge dismissing special-ist knowledge) or inability to establish a proper interaction with professionals concerning explanations about the child's disorder (declaring a 'no relation to knowledge') is basically related, from the point of view of social affective positions, to the motionless statement of leading a difficult life. These features, that pair with blurred positions regarding etiologic and therapeutic concep-tions, reveal *'letting go logic'* associated with an underprivileged social condi-tion. This letting go approach characterizes ambivalence of thought and absence of construction of an explanatory model of the child's disorder that is likely to open up to some form of action.

Discussion

Our approach to 'negative public attitudes' has been encompassed from the point of view of therapeutic relationship as told by parents of adolescents who, during their childhood, have shown signs of psychological problems and have been treated by a pluridisciplinary team at the Day Center in Lausanne. Our approach also includes two supplementary viewpoints: (1) criteria for assessing clinicians and special education teachers and (2) the way parents talk about their references to knowledge required in order to understand the child's problem – their own knowledge as well as the specialist's knowledge, the way in which they talk about disruptions in their life resulting from the child's problem, and how they adopted a position – either as actors or agents – as regards their child's treatment.

We treated the theme of distance between 'scientific' knowledge and lay knowledge by identifying the parents' structural pattern connected both with the etiology of the disorder and trends in therapeutics, and liable to be compat-ible or antagonistic with the two main theoretical trends that have successively prevailed in the course of the history of psychiatric and medical thought: the biomedical and social psychological model.

The problem arising from both themes, 'negative attitudes' and 'distance between knowledge', is obviously their mutual reduction; reducing distance could affect negative attitudes. But is it so simple? If this was the case, the outlet would then be to promote public information campaigns based on psychiatric theoretical conceptions and means of treatment. Our research questions the belief that it is possible to 'educate' people and to track down the 'appropriate teaching methods'. It shows that the problem is by far more complex. Success of a therapeutic approach lies in the relationship and com-munication between different forms of knowledge. Doubtlessly our research was pursued in a limited and set environment: 52 professionals for 32 families with a particular characteristic: their child had been diagnosed as having a psychological disorder. But, considering the more qualitative investigation, analyzing a limited number of cases can unclose more general reflections.

Does this put off the question of informing the public? Or course not, but an information campaign should encompass didactic transposition and not be conceived as dispatching 'proper' knowledge likely to replace 'inaccurate' knowledge.

Therapists should appreciate that all knowledge is elaborated from preexisting conceptions and knowledge that should be taken into consideration and therefore unveiled. This is far from simple as it implies investigating in detail how people relate to illness, to their body, to standards and identifying the family and social settings where disorders are detected, declared and produced.

All factors, contributing to the gradual emergence of meanings connected with the causes of the child's problem and ways to treat them, produced by people consulting therapists, should then be taken into consideration. Consequently this means that therapists have to tackle various intricate dimensions with a dynamic perspective such as the way consultants conceive their own relations to knowledge and the various valorizations comprised both in the general social environment and in the social group where various stages of socialization operate and are pursued. They also have to question how they imagine their accountability or their subjection to a determinism they cannot escape: at the same time representations influence their ability to react to strains that affect the course of their own life and to achieve cooperation with other specialists, eventually in situations of conflicting dynamics.

Conclusion

All communication takes place within an interaction where representations of oneself and of other partners are constantly negotiated. Our data testify that interactive processes of constructing these representations are socially connoted. People from the most privileged social conditions settle in to negotiating knowledge with specialists according to actor logic and as an active reaction against disruption; these people also develop conceptions close to a social psychological model of etiology and therapeutics. People from the most underprivileged social conditions display the 'letting go' attitude: they believe that they do not have any form of knowledge likely to be integrated into the course of contacts with a therapist, nor that they are in any way partners in an appropriate remediation both for their child and for the consequences of this problem in the course of their own life. Representations of etiology and therapeutics remain blurry and unorganized.

As for most professionals, they are unfortunately prone to thinking that a therapeutic encounter is based on the patient's problem regarding his physical and psychological health, on one hand, and on specialized knowledge and techniques considered suitable in order to decode the patient's message and to treat it, on the other hand. This attitude bypasses the fact that efficiency is instantly connected with a first identification of the patient's cooperation, opposition or letting go dispositions. It also implies discarding the fact that disparities in social positioning are also involved in the interaction between patient and specialist and, therefore, inflect these dispositions.

Enabling parents, accustomed to medical care, to express themselves in the course of the research of the social representations of their child's disorder also offers a unique opportunity to really listen to them. One of the mothers said so in the following words: 'I think that just doing research and listening to us is something ... I hope this research will help improve things ... especially in dealing with clients!' But their words will only be heard when professionals in effect take into consideration the social logic that inflects possibilities of treating emotions, negotiating knowledge and handling action.

References

1 Cramer B: La psychiatrie expliquée: une mission impossible? Cah Psychiatr Genevois 1991;11:7–13.
2 Duruz N, Schurmans MN, Lob R, Martinez E, Seferdjeli L: Les représentations sociales de la maladie mentale de l'enfant. Rapport au fonds National de la Recherche Scientifique Suisse, Berne, 1997.
3 Lebart L, Salem A: Statistique textuelle. Paris, Dunod, 1994.
4 Cibois PH: Le PEM, pourcentage de l'écart maximum: un indice de liaison entre modalités d'un tableau de contingence. Bull Méthodol Sociol 1993;40:43–63.
5 Cibois PH: L'analyse factorielle. Paris, Presses Universitaires de France, 1994.
6 Laplantine F: Anthropologie de la maladie. Paris, Payot, 1986.
7 Dufrancatel C: La sociologie des maladies mentales. Sociol Contemp 1968;16:2.
8 Herzlich C: Sante et maladie. Analyse d'une représentation sociale. Paris-La Haye, Mouton, 1969.
9 Herzlich C: Médecine, maladie et société. Paris-La Haye, Mouton, 1970.
10 Herzlich C: Perceptions et représentations des usagers. Santé, corps, handicap; in Conceptions, mesures et actions en santé publique. Paris, INSERM, 1982.
11 Herzlich C: Représentations sociales de la santé et de la maladie et leur dynamique dans le champ social; in Doise W, Palmonari A (eds): L'Etude des représentations sociales. Neuchâtel Delachaux Niestlé, 1986, pp 157–170.
12 Schurmans MN: Maladie mentale et sens commun. Une étude de sociologie de la connaissance. Neuchâtel, Delachaux Niestlé, 1990.

Marie-Noëlle Schurmans, Faculté de Psychologie et des Sciences de l'Education,
Université de Genève, Route de Drize, 9, CH–1227 Carouge (Switzerland)
Tel. +41 22 705 96 24, Fax +41 22 342 89 24

Guimón J, Fischer W, Sartorius N (eds): The Image of Madness. The Public Facing Mental Illness and Psychiatric Treatment. Basel, Karger, 1999, pp 85–95

········· ·················

Differentiating between the Professions of Psychologists and Psychiatrists: A Field Study in Vizcaya

Luis Yllá, María S. Hidalgo

Department of Neuroscience, University of the Basque Country, School of Medicine, Bilbao, Spain

Although psychiatrists and psychologists – particularly in their clinical speciality – work together in mental health centers, their role is not sufficiently differentiated for the general public to have a clear idea of the roles played by these two professions. In fact, throughout our experience as professionals in psychology and psychiatry and, indeed, as individuals belonging to a specific population group – in this case, the city of Bilbao – we have found that the population in question is frequently confused about the professional roles of the psychologist and the psychiatrist, and often has difficulty in deciding which of the two professionals to turn to in cases of specific problems or ailments. The fact that there are also fields in which the tasks of both professions are combined (e.g. psychotherapy) adds even more to the confusion.

On the other hand, there are also other professions offering psychological help. Greenblatt [1] reports that in a population of people with problems and mental disorders, 42% consulted priests, 29% general practitioners, 18 % psychiatrists or psychologists and 10% various other official organizations. Of all these, 58% felt they had received suitable assistance.

The relationship between psychiatry and clinical psychology has been changing at the same rate as the latter has become organized as a professional discipline and has taken on the task of diagnosis and evaluation, of therapies and behavioral changes as well as the appraisal of results and investigation. This has not been an easy task and it has been said that psychology in general, and clinical psychology in particular, has undergone a crisis and a devaluation in recent years motivated primarily by the intense biologization of psychiatry.

Psychiatry has also been changing over the last few decades and, as Guimón [2] says, it finds itself at a crossroads. It is not surprising, therefore, that its public image is in the process of changing as reported by Lamontagne [3] who believes that the image of the psychiatrist goes hand in hand with the image of psychiatry and in particular with the role of the psychiatrist as an educator of the public.

Chung and Prasher [4] in a study among students did not find differences between males and females when they were asked about the image they had of psychiatrists and, in any case, the image improved after a course in psychiatry at the university. In fact, the image that people have of the psychiatrist depends on various factors, sometimes only indirectly related to psychiatry as, for example, the stereotypes of the psychiatrist portrayed in the films which Clara describes [5]. But in any case there is no doubt that responsibility for the public image of psychiatrists rests with psychiatrists themselves, as has been reported by Bourne [6] in 1978.

In Spain, one of the most documented studies is that of Ruiz Ruiz [7] who showed that, in the late 1970s, the attitudes of the population towards the psychiatrist were mainly negative and in direct relation to people's ignorance about mental diseases. If a family member suffered from a nervous condition, 76% would tend to consult a general practitioner and only 23% a psychiatrist. Of those interviewed, 34% had visited a psychiatrist at some time, either themselves or a member of their family, and 40% believed that they should only consult a psychiatrist as a last resort. The upper social classes were more likely to consult a psychiatrist, whereas 70% of cases in the lower class did not consider the psychiatrist necessary. Of the professional groups, those most likely to consult a psychiatrist if they had a psychological problem were health sector employees (68%) and business people (62%) while those least likely to consult a psychiatrist were in the legal and religious professions (15 and 20%, respectively).

In a study that we carried out among the population of Vizcaya [8], we were able to show that the image of psychiatry and attitudes towards the mentally ill was quite negative and authoritarian in general.

More recently, it has been shown in a study by Guimón [2] that 16% of the family members of students in their final years of medicine or newly qualified doctors who had chosen the speciality of psychiatry were unhappy with the choice of the student/doctor, which indicates that even in the 1990s there are many people with a low opinion of psychiatrists and their speciality.

Materials and Methods

In the context of a wider study, we tried to define the image that the population of Vizcaya has of the psychologist and the psychiatrist. This field research was carried out among the general population of Vizcaya, using 400 structured interviews in a random sample, stratified proportionally according to age, sex and residence by means of the random route system, to represent the population aged 16–65. The information was gathered during an uninterrupted 3-week period. The statistical error ranges from ±5% with a confidence level of 95%. Interviews were also conducted independently among all five classes of psychology students at the Deusto University (565 students) with the statistical error ranging from ±2.4% and a confidence level also of 95%. All the analyses were performed with SPSS. The survey was designed and conducted by us.

Results

Professional Help for Marital Difficulties

When asked 'Who would you go to for professional help if you had marital difficulties?' 1 out of 4 people ruled out any help, either because they would not go to anyone (19.8%) or because they would not know where to go (5.5%). Forty-four percent, however, would choose a psychologist if they found themselves in that situation. The rest of the options lag far behind; neither priests (5%) nor doctors (4.5%) nor psychiatrists (2.5%) attain the levels of confidence that people place in psychologists.

There is a significant relationship between seeking professional help for marital problems and professional occupation. Homemakers clearly chose the psychologist (52.1%), while relatively few students would tend to go to a psychologist (34.2%), trying to solve this kind of problem alone (26.6%) more often than members of other occupations. A relation was found between the socioeconomic standing one enjoys and the confidence one places in psychologists; as standing rises, confidence in psychologists sinks, and the tendency grows in the high status bracket. Marital status also influences one's choice of professional help. Almost half the married sample (49.4%) chose a psychologist for this kind of problem. In the unmarried, the proportion was smaller, 1 out of 3 (34.3%). Age makes a significant difference in how one goes about finding help. From the age of 51 up, the classic figures of the priest and the doctor were relied upon at a rate above the population's average. Though the percentage of persons who would go to the psychologist was high for all ages, at the threshold of maturity (ages 41–50), the tendency was sharper. Interestingly, among those people who had professional contact with a psychologist, 50% would go to a psychologist for marriage guidance, a percentage much higher than for the general population.

Seeking Help for Depression

When asked what they would do about depression, more than 8 out of 10 surveyed would accept professional help. The psychologist was the choice of 38.8% of those surveyed, outdistancing the classic alternative of the doctor (11%) and even more so, the psychiatrist (7%).

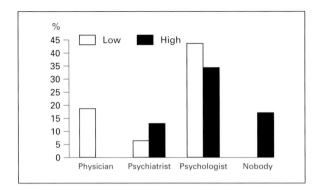

Fig. 1. Socioeconomic status and people who would seek some kind of help.

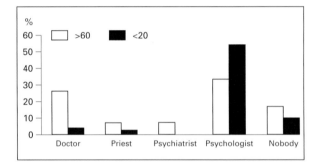

Fig. 2. Age and search for help.

Forty-eight percent of the time, women would choose a psychologist to cope with depression, while men, on the other hand, would do so only 30% of the time. Many men would take other unconventional routes (28.4%), and 20% of all men would not go to anyone. For depression, men would tend to seek less psychological help than women, but such differences disappeared for other kinds of professionals (doctors, priests and psychiatrists). Generally speaking, students (44.3%) and homemakers (43.7%) may be said to be the groups most likely to choose psychologists. Homemakers displayed an above average percentage in their tendency to go to the doctor as well (14.3%).

According to figure 1, which analyzes the socioeconomic status, the lower the socioeconomic status, the higher the percentage of people who would seek some kind of help, while people of a high status display the greatest reluctance to do so. Thus, 43.5% of the low-status subjects would go to a psychologist, and 18.8% to the doctor. In contrast, high-status survey subjects would prefer to place themselves in the hands of a psychiatrist (13%).

Table 1. Proportion of use of psychologists and psychiatrists by higher socioeconomic status holders compared to the general population (%)

	Psychologist	Psychiatrist
Mid-high	31.5	14.8
High	34.8	13
Total population	38.8	7

Table 2. Proportion of nonusers of help according to the socioeconomic status (%)

	Low	Mid-low	Middle	Mid-high	High
Nonuser	0.0	12.4	16.9	18.5	17.4

Higher socioeconomic status holders show a lower tendency to use psychologists and a higher tendency to use psychiatrists than the average population (table 1). Furthermore, as the socioeconomic status rises, the population tends to shy away from any kind of help at all (table 2). Single persons are more apt to seek unconventional help (30.7%) and are also the least likely to go to their doctor. On the age question (see figure 2), there is a contrast between young adults and senior citizens in the hypothetical search for help. Young adults are characterized by going almost exclusively to the psychologist (53.8%). Senior citizens display greater independence from the outside world and would go to their doctors (26.2%) who become more important as subjects age, the although the subjects would not rule out other kinds of help, such as psychiatrists or priests. Fifty-three percent of those who have gone to a psychologist at some time would go to the psychologist to cope with this kind of problem.

Difference between a Psychologist and a Psychiatrist
A large portion of the population sees a difference between psychologists and psychiatrists, although in the answers given, 14% either did not know or did not answer, 5% saw no difference, and 30.5% catalogued one of the professionals but did not differentiate it from the other ('Psychiatrists treat serious problems', 'I feel more confident with psychologists' or 'Psychologists

Table 3. Differentiation between psychologist and psychiatrist

	n	%
Psychiatrists treat serious problems (madness, nerves)	10	26.1
Psychiatrists handle mental illness and psychologists handle day-to-day problems	86	21
Psychiatrists are doctors who can prescribe drugs, psychologists aren't	68	16.5
Psychiatrists treat physical problems, and psychologists treat behavior	25	6.1
They're similar, they both help people	20	4.9
I feel more confident with a psychologist	11	2.7
Psychologists are for children	7	1.7
Other	29	7.1
I don't know	50	12.2
No answer	7	1.7
Total	410	100.0

are for children', table 3). In these cases, the function of the psychiatrist was more clearly defined (26.1%), while 5% of the answers did not refer to psychologists.

The psychiatrist was described as having a medical role (treatment of physical disturbances, mental illness, prescription-giving power), while the psychologist was associated with day-to-day problems and behavior, outside the health care system and assigned the role of a counselor.

Primary Motivation for Consulting a Psychologist

When asked about the primary motivation of a person going to the psychologist, 1 out of 3 people felt that one should go to the psychologist for nervous problems, except for those who believed one should go for personal problems (18.3%) or emotional problems (15.3%). The educational facet was associated less with psychology (6.3%). Nevertheless, only 4% of the population rejected the idea of someone going to the psychologist.

Table 4 shows the relationship between socioeconomic status and the reasons why people go to the psychologist, although it is a trifle confusing, since emotional problems and nervous problems are the same, and it is difficult for surveyors to establish what people mean when they make such a distinction.

Reasons for Consulting a Psychiatrist

For 3 out of 4 people, the reasons for which a person should go to the psychiatrist were medical (77.8%). In 52.5% of these cases, the reasons were

Table 4. Reasons for consulting a psychologist according to the socioeconomic status (%)

	Low	Mid-high	High	Total population
Personal problems	12.5	7.4	17.4	18.3
Emotional problems	25	14	17.4	15.3
Nervous problems	43.8	46.3	17.4	34.5

Table 5. Proportion of people linking madness to psychiatrists according to the socioeconomic status (%)

	Low	Mid-low	Middle	Mid-high	High	Total population
Madness	56.3	59.2	49.2	46.3	30.4	52.5

related with madness, and in 25.3% with illness. Visits for other reasons were unimportant; most of the population focused on these two aspects. Rejection of the psychiatrist barely reached 4%, though the classic literary image pigeonholing psychiatrists with the mentally unbalanced persists.

Low-status persons predominated among those who did not know why a person should go to a psychiatrist (25% of the low-status population). High-status subjects related the psychiatrist mainly with illness (34.8%) and were the least likely to relate the psychiatrist with madness. The analysis of the relationship between psychiatrists and madness shows that this is an established relationship (table 5). Psychiatrists were identified with illness by an average of 25.3% of the population and with madness by 52.5%.

Confidence in Psychological and Psychiatric Services

In the event of needing to go to a psychiatrist or a psychologist, the population answered as follows: 'I would go to the psychologist' 39%, 'I would go to the psychiatrist' 9%, 'I wouldn't go to either' 15.8%, 'I wouldn't know who to go to' 12.3%, and 'I would go to either one' 24%.

Students would trust the psychologist (48.1%) more than the rest of the population, while homemakers were the group that showed least trust (17.6%). As for socioeconomic status (see fig. 3), higher-status levels preferred the psychiatrist, and had the smallest percentage of trust in the psychologist. Low-status holders, however, were the least distrustful, and 93.7% of them would choose to go to either or both.

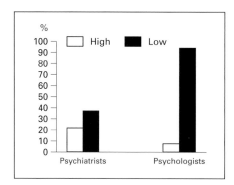

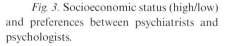

Fig. 3. Socioeconomic status (high/low) and preferences between psychiatrists and psychologists.

The psychologist was also the professional least likely to be chosen by the unmarried (47.4%). Unmarried persons with marital status other than single (divorced, separated or widowed) mistrusted either professional to a greater extent (22.2%) than the average of the population (15.8%). Up until the age of 30, people place more trust in the psychologist. Mature persons (41–60) chose both. Regarding those aged 60, the percentage of people who did not know increased considerably (23.8%), but their confidence in the psychologist may also be seen to be smaller and their confidence in the psychiatrist greater than that of other age groups. One of every 2 people who had consulted a psychologist would trust a psychologist in case of need, and they would trust either profession more than persons who had no experience with psychologists. The same was true among those who knew a psychologist personally, that is, they trusted psychologists more and had a lower percentage of 'I don't know'/'no answer'.

Perception of the Function of Psychologists

When establishing the function of the psychologist, by far the most widespread view was that psychologists dealt with healthy people who had psychological and social problems (60.8%). It should be stressed that it was people with a low socioeconomic standing who mostly (75%) related the psychologist with healthy people who had problems. As far as age goes, for almost 7 out of 10 young adults (under 30), the psychologist was the person who treated healthy people with psychological or social problems. This proportion decreased at higher ages. Thus, a much lower percentage of senior citizens (over 60) identified the psychologist with healthy persons than in the population as a whole; the elderly were more apt to relate the psychologist with the treatment of the sick in general than all other age groups (19%), as they placed the medical function in the lead (table 6).

Table 6. Proportion of people identifying psychologists as therapists for both healthy or ill persons according to age (%)

	Age groups						Total population
	<20	21–30	31–40	41–50	51–60	>60	
Healthy with problems	71.2	66.3	53.8	64.1	58.6	47.6	60.8
Ill	5.8	2.2	7.5	4.7	5.7	19	6.5

The Differences between Psychology and Psychiatry as Perceived by Psychology Students at the Deusto University

A certain difficulty is frequently found in differentiating between the psychologist and the psychiatrist. This is why we decided to see to what extent psychology students were aware of these differences. We offered them four possibilities: type of people: The psychologist deals with normal people who have problems, and the psychiatrist deals with the mentally ill; approach: the psychologist uses a psychological approach, and the psychiatrist uses a pharmacological one; seriousness of the mental illness: the psychiatrist deals with the more seriously mentally ill. I see no difference between the two disciplines. As may be seen in figure 4, most students believed that the difference lay in the approach (74.3%). The next most frequent criterion regarding the difference was the type of people who would go to psychologists and psychiatrists (13.3%).

Discussion

We conducted a study of the distinction made by the population of Vizcaya between psychologists and psychiatrists and, on the assumption that there might be some differences of interest, we compared our sample of the general population with psychology students at the University of Deusto (Bilbao, Vizcaya). The overall results are thus outlined to indicate the few differences of emphasis.

Psychology students clearly differentiate the role of the psychologist from that of the psychiatrist with the majority stating that these differences lie basically in the approach adopted: drugs by psychiatrists and exclusively psychological therapies by psychologists. These opinions are consistent throughout the group though of course unawareness is greater among students in earlier courses.

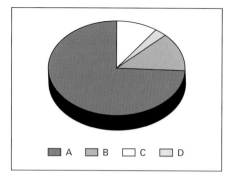

Fig. 4. Differences students describe between psychologists and psychiatrists. A = Approach; B = type of people; C = seriousness of the mental illness; D = I see no differences.

Knowledge of what constitutes a psychologist and the associated acceptance is improving significantly in our context and is even winning ground from psychiatrists. The psychologist is specifically identified as someone who helps to 'solve problems', thereby associating psychologists more with the healthy than with the mentally ill. On the other hand, those from a lower social-cultural context would, in proportion, be more likely to consult a psychologist while those from higher classes would tend, if necessary, to visit a psychiatrist. In our system, psychiatrists enjoy a higher social standing and they are more expensive than psychologists, which undoubtedly explains the difference to which we refer.

Psychologists tend to be more likely consulted for depression probably because, in Spain, the word 'depression' has been popularized to the extent that it no longer bears the serious connotations it so frequently has and is also used as a catchall category to refer to any nervous disorder as a situational problem: we think this coincides with the idea of the psychologist as one who helps to resolve problems. Women more often prefer psychological procedures over those doctors are assumed to use and we believe that this is probably because women in general are more open to their 'inner lives' than men and so have a greater capacity for insight.

Precisely because the students are studying psychology, they tend to choose professionals from their field; this is accentuated by the fact that, in this country, even at university level, psychologists are involved in some kind of class struggle with psychiatrists.

Because courses in psychology are relatively new here, it is hardly surprising that older people are more likely to consult doctors, particularly those who are not psychiatrists, because of a degree of scepticism which has always been felt toward the latter. On the other hand, the fact that those who have used the services of a psychologist at some time tend to place a greater value on them suggests that these professionals are indeed offering a good service, gradually winning prestige in this country.

Conclusion

The distinction the population makes between psychiatrists and psychologists was investigated in a research study carried out among the population of Vizcaya with 400 structured interviews in a random sample, stratified proportionally according to age, sex and residence to represent the Viscaya population aged 16–65. 43.5% of the low-status survey subjects would go to psychologists, and 18.8% to the doctor. In counterpoint high-status subjects would prefer to place themselves in the hands of a psychiatrist (13%) and showed lesser use of a psychologist. Young adults are characterized by going almost exclusively to the psychologist. The psychiatrist in comparison is given a medical role (treatment of physical disturbances, mental illness, prescription-giving power) and is identified with madness and illness, while the psychologist is associated with day-to-day problems and behavior, outside the health care system and assigned the role of a counselor.

References

1   Greenblatt M: Papel del profesional de salud mental comunitaria; in Freedman AM, Kaplan HI, Sadock BJ (eds): Tratado de Psiquiatría. Barcelona, Salvat, 1982, vol 2, pp 2599–2604.
2   Guimón J: Psiquiatras: De brujos a burócratas. Barcelona, Salvat, 1990.
3   Lamontagne Y: The public image of psychiatrists. Can J Psychiatry 1990;35:693–695.
4   Chung MG, Prasher VP: Differences in attitudes among medical students towards psychiatry in one English university. Psychol Rep 1995;77:843–847.
5   Clara A: The image of the psychiatrist in motion pictures. Acta Psychiatr Belg 1995;95:7–15.
6   Bourne PG: The psychiatrist's responsibility and the public trust. Am J Psychiatry 1978;135:174–177.
7   Ruiz Ruiz M: La imagen de la locura. Barcelona, CEPYP, 1979.
8   Yllá L, Ozámis A, Guimón J: Un análisis psicosocial de las actitudes hacia el enfermo mental. Madrid, Asociación española de Neuropsiquiatria. Colección monográfica. Premios nacionales, 1981.

Prof. Luis Yllá, Departamento de Neurociencias, Seccion Psiquiatría,
Universidad del País Vasco (UPV),
E–48940 Lejona, Vizcaya (Spain)
Tel./Fax +34 44 436 488

Guimón J, Fischer W, Sartorius N (eds): The Image of Madness. The Public Facing Mental Illness and Psychiatric Treatment. Basel, Karger, 1999, pp 96–104

••••••••••••••••••••••••

One of the Last Obstacles to Better Mental Health Care: The Stigma of Mental Illness

Norman Sartorius

Department of Psychiatry, University Hospital, Geneva, Switzerland

The quality of mental health care can be judged by a number of criteria. From the point of view of the patients, care is of a good quality if access to it is unrestricted, if they are treated with respect, if they receive unbiased, well-documented and comprehensible information about treatment options likely to be useful in their case and if they can express their preference for any of them, if treatment is provided with the necessary expertise avoiding any possible harm and maximizing its benefits, if the information about them and their illness is kept confidential, if they can afford the cost of the care that they receive without severe restrictions of other needs, and if their human rights are respected during the treatment process.

From the point of view of the medical profession care is of a good quality if it is provided by a qualified person, if it is given in appropriate surroundings, if there are sufficient evidence and experience about the effectiveness and safety of the methods that are being proposed, if a relationship of trust and respect can be established between the patient and the personnel providing treatment, if the rights and requirements of the staff working in mental health facilities are respected, and if the evaluation of the quality of care is done in a transparent and well-documented way.

The authorities that are responsible for the provision of mental health care judge the quality of care by comparing what is done with the rules and standards established on the basis of evidence and experience. To assess it, authorities have to define indicators of quality. These include indicators of input in terms of investment into health care, of process in terms of flow of the operation, of output in terms of numbers of interventions performed, of outcome in terms of changes of the states of health of individuals or communities, and of impact in terms of consequences that the health care intervention had for the health service and society in a broader sense. For each of these indicators, there is a qualitative (how well) and a quantitative (how much) reply.

The stigma of mental illness affects every one of the above requirements for care of a good quality. Access to care will depend on the perception of the illness by the authorities and by the general population. If people with mental illness are perceived as dangerous, lazy, unreliable, unemployable and unlikely to ever recover from their condition there will be much opposition to the placement of mental health facilities in low-crime neighborhoods, in buildings of good quality, within easy reach by means of public transport, and in operation in, say, evening hours.

Access also depends on the ability to pay: the stigma of mental illness reduces the willingness of authorities to provide financial resources that would allow the provision of care of a good quality to all people who suffer from mental illness and they themselves often do not have sufficient money to spend on getting the best possible treatment. The consequence is that they are denied access to the best care and that services of a lower quality are offered often with considerable administrative expenditure. Suboptimal care has poorer results, which confirms the myth of the untreatability of mental illness; it also enhances the feeling of not having a fair deal of both the patients and the professionals who are responsible for providing the treatment. Poor working conditions also affect the quality of applicants for the positions in the mental health system: although undoubtedly such conditions are seen as a challenge and are attractive to a certain proportion of candidates entering the profession, most of those driven by a mixture of material and idealistic motives in their choice of profession hesitate and finally choose another discipline or field of work in medicine. Insufficient resources reduce the range of treatment methods offered (which diminishes the patients' options in choosing treatments) and make it difficult for professionals active in the field to upgrade or update their knowledge and skills through additional training. Paradoxically, the stigma of mental illness having contributed to the poorer quality of the service also contributes to the smaller likelihood that information about the patients and their diseases will be protected against being divulged to others.

Stigma of Mental Illness Is Ubiquitous and Growing

Stigma is attached to mental illness in all societies. Sometimes it leads to positive discrimination as for example in situations in which symptoms of mental illness are interpreted as being an indication of a divine possession of the individual who is so marked. Most often, however, stigma results in a negative discrimination of the person who has the illness. Usually the discrimination does not stop there: stigma and discrimination also affect the person's family, in the present and across generations. The stigma attached to mental illness and negative discrimination also spread to the health services – mental hospitals, psychotropic drugs, psychiatrists and other mental health personnel; in general, it is pervasive and detrimental.

Stigma and intolerance of differences (and in particular the differences that may be the result of mental illness) have grown in recent decades. Several factors might be responsible for this. Urbanization, for example by increasing population density in towns, makes it more probable that people will not be able (or willing) to tolerate in their immediate neighborhood anyone who on occasion or frequently displays disturbing behavior. The growing complexity of labor makes it less probable that people who are less well qualified or lost qualifications because of impairments produced by illness will find employment; this in turn has a negative influence on their health and contributes to the stigma that they bear. The media have over many years (and more intrusively in recent years because of their growing power) presented a negative image of those suffering from mental illness. Villains in television dramas and films are very often shown to be mentally abnormal or sick. Violent behavior is portrayed as an almost certain indication of mental illness (although most of the violence is perpetrated by people who have never suffered from any form of diagnosable mental disorder). Mental health services are presented in the media and in art with a bias underlining their dark and negative features, compared with other types of health services which are shown to do a lot of valuable work. There are of course in the history of psychiatry many reasons for negative opinions about mental illness and the systems in which people suffering from it had to live with their illness. Although many of these reasons have disappeared – today it is possible for example to provide effective treatment and protect the human rights of the mentally ill much better than ever before – the mental health services retain their negative image, which is further reinforced by their presentation in the media, arts and writings of antipsychiatric groups. The growth of the proportion of middle class citizens in many countries contributes to the stabilization and standardization of behavior and to the reluctance to make exceptions and tolerate difference. The interpenetration of cultures – noticeably worldwide – also seems to be finding its expression in an amazing and increasing similarity of dress, preferences for music and food, modes of entertainment and leisure activities, which makes the life of those who are somewhat different much more difficult.

Table 1. Cycle of disadvantage: points of intervention

Steps to disadvantage	Interventions
Disease	Prevention or recovery through treatment
Impairment	Correction of impairment
Stigma linked to disease or impairment	Disassociation of stigma and disease (or impairment)
Discrimination linked to stigma	Reduction of discrimination even if stigma persists
Reduction of opportunities for rehabilitation	Adding options for employment and performance in new social roles
Role malfunction enhancing disease and impairment	Destigmatization of role malfunction

Breaking the Cycle of Disadvantage

Breaking the cycle of disadvantage resulting from stigma is clearly a priority. Recent reports [1] indicate that mental disorders are responsible for a major proportion of all disability in the world and that there are indications that this situation will deteriorate. Reports from a multitude of studies [2] show that treatment of mental disorders is possible, effective and low in cost. Well-developed mental health programs could help those who are mentally ill and their families: at present neither treatment nor care is available for the majority of people who would benefit from it. In the developing countries (but also elsewhere) resources available for mental health services are minimal and the situations described above reduce the likelihood that psychiatric services and mental health programs in general will receive a higher priority unless resolute action is taken. Table 1 indicates the steps in the cycle of disadvantage: at each of them interventions might be effective and should be attempted.

In the instance of psychiatry primary prevention of disorders is possible for a variety of disorders of a known pathogenesis. A striking example for the possibility of primary prevention is cretinism due to iodine deficiency in the mothers' food: the correction of this deficiency would drastically reduce the incidence of a serious form of mental impairment. The role of psychiatrists in this intervention is to advocate public health measures that will have to be implemented by other parts of the health service system – a role that would be similar in a number of other primary prevention interventions [3].

For a number of other psychiatric disorders the possibilities of prevention are limited or nonexistent: in these instances successful treatment can reduce the duration of the abnormal state, reduce impairment and increase the similarity of the psychiatric disorders to other diseases. Where treatment possibilities are limited and therefore impairment cannot be prevented or the disease lasts for a longer time the interventions should focus on the diminution of the stigma linked to the disease – by health education, media action, appropriate training of health personnel and other measures. In a number of instances it will not be possible to separate the disease from its stigma: where this is the case, public health interventions will have to be joined with legal interventions to reduce and eventually eliminate the negative discrimination linked to the stigmatized disease and persons who suffer from it. Stigma and discrimination diminish possibilities of rehabilitation and of normal functioning in various social and personal roles: the next level of intervention will therefore be oriented to the development of new and added options of employment and involvement of individuals suffering from mental disorders. Finally, in some instances prevention will not be possible and the disease will lead to an impairment and a considerable reduction of quality of performance in various social roles ranging from employment and parenting to self-care and avoiding harm: in these instances the interventions will have to be directed to the disassociation of the malfunction and the negative discrimination that might be caused by such malfunction.

The decision to make a major investment of resources into the disruption of the cycle of disadvantage described above is both conceptual and practical. The concept of a mental disorder as a lasting condition that is always marked by significant impairments of personal and social functioning will have to be modified: both health care staff and the general public including people with mental illness should, for example, accept the notion that mental illness is not always of long duration; that an episode of illness does not mean that the person who experienced it should thenceforth be considered as mentally ill; that most mental disorders do not involve significant disruptions of role performance and even when they do that role performance can be reestablished to previous levels; that the behavior of most people in society is not perfect and that it is therefore both just and reasonable to be tolerant to aberrations of behavior and nonconformist lifestyles; that being employed and economically productive are neither the only nor the most important signs of mental health; that in instances of a comorbidity between mental and physical disorders both conditions should be treated; and that the treatment of mental disorders significantly improves the prognosis of the physical disorder and vice versa.

In harmony with conceptual modifications it will also be necessary to reexamine the manner in which psychiatric treatment is being planned and provided. In addition to the obvious need for respect for the patient and the protection of his or her rights it is also important to give preference to treatments that do not contribute to the stigmatization of the illness; the patient should, for example, be treated in the general health facilities rather than in mental institutions of sinister reputation and treatments should be chosen that do not produce visible side effects (or doses should be adjusted to minimize such side effects even if this means that the reduction of psychiatric symptoms is slower or incomplete). It is also necessary to reexamine the relationship between doctor and patient: taking time and paying careful attention to patients' descriptions of ways in which they used to overcome or live with their disease, for example, will provide the doctor with valuable new knowledge that can be conveyed to other patients and used in the training of psychiatrists, general practitioners and other health staff.

Programs Aiming to Reduce Stigma and Discrimination Resulting from Mental Illness

The fact that the stigma and discrimination resulting from mental illness are among the main obstacles to providing mental health care of an appropriate quality is being recognized in a number of countries and in some of them, e.g. United Kingdom or Australia, campaigns against this stigma have been undertaken by the governments or nongovernmental organizations.

The World Psychiatric Association (WPA) has also initiated an international program to fight the stigma and discrimination resulting from schizophrenia. Schizophrenia has been selected as a focus for this program for several reasons. It is a severe mental illness with symptoms that people usually associate with mental illness – such as hallucinations, delusions (often of a bizarre and incomprehensible kind), psychomotor abnormalities and incoherence of speech. The disorder is often of a long duration and can produce impairments of various kinds. Rehabilitation after the illness can be difficult and to large extent depends on the attitudes and behavior of people surrounding the patients and of the patients themselves. It was felt that reducing the stigma related to schizophrenia is a particularly challenging task but that success of this program would significantly improve the quality of life of people who have schizophrenia (and of those who care for them) and could help in developing similar programs for other diseases.

The program which the WPA started differs from others in several ways. First, it is international and has global drive. Next, it is organized in a cumulative fashion: the experience obtained in the first country in which it is employed is made available to the groups starting it in the second country, both of these will serve as a source of inspiration and experience for the third country and so on. The program was started in the province of Alberta in Canada; programs in an urban area in Spain and in a province in Austria were initiated in 1999 and it is expected that before August 1999 at least eight countries will have programs underway. The program is directed by a Steering Committee[1] that coordinates the action in the different countries as well as the production of program material and action tools.

The WPA program does not approach the problem of discrimination and stigma in a blunderbuss manner shooting messages at all people at the same time: it is selective, targeting interventions at groups likely to be important in the process of attitude change. It does not start with theory: it begins the program with an exploration of the experience of people who suffer from schizophrenia and gives priority to the elimination of specific problems that have been causing distress to them. The program is not conducted by psychiatrists: rather, psychiatrists are trying to be helpful members of the group that does it. These groups include representatives of different community organizations, experts in different disciplines, members of patient and family organizations, journalists, politicians and others. A central notion of the program is that the achievable is more attractive than the ideal. Where stigma cannot be rapidly removed for example, the program seeks to diminish discrimination as a result of the disease, as a first step; where discrimination is difficult to fight and overcome the program focuses on providing alternatives to situations in which discrimination is particularly harmful or painful.

Support for the program comes from different sources. An unrestricted educational grant from Eli Lilly helped to start the work and supports the process of developing of material for the program. Local support comes from governmental and nongovernmental organizations, industrial and individual donations. None of those working on the program receive a salary: the reward lies in the feeling of being involved in a noble and necessary enterprise.

The material that has been produced so far includes a step-by-step description of the activities that should be undertaken in each of the countries participating in the program. An estimate of time is given for each of the steps: it is, however, recognized that countries might vary in the amount of time they need to accomplish each of the steps. There is also a description of schizophrenia summarizing knowledge about the disorder and indicating facts that are of particular importance for programs aiming

[1] The members of the Steering Committee are Prof. N. Sartorius (Chairman) Prof. J.J. Lopez-lbor, Prof. C. Stefanis and Prof. N.N. Wig.

to diminish stigma and discrimination as a result of mental illness. These two documents, the Guidelines for Programme Development [4] and the Summary of Knowledge about Schizophrenia developed for the WPA Program against Stigma and Discrimination because of Schizophrenia [4] have been developed by working groups composed of experts from different countries representing different disciplines likely to be a source of useful information for the program. Three further documents are being developed: a description of the program development in each of the places that participate in the first phase of the program (volume 3), a description of similar or related programs that have been undertaken in the past (volume 4) and a 'tool kit' containing material that could be useful to those developing programs e.g. videotapes, posters, films and books (volume 5). Each of the materials included in volume 5 was evaluated by a special review group and is accompanied by a brief note suggesting when, how and where the material could be used.

Once the first group of countries has completed their work the program will be released for general use. Some of the experts who participated in the development of the program material and those who conducted the program in the first eight places will be available as advisors for groups or countries that will undertake the program in the future. The programs in the first eight places will, however, continue and it is expected that an evaluation of the effects of the program will be undertaken again after several years.

Conclusions

Stigma attached to mental illness and the negative discrimination that is usually associated with stigmatization are significant obstacles to the development of mental health programs. They can be diminished and perhaps even avoided. Work in this field is of primary importance for mental health programs and for psychiatry as a discipline. Relevant activities have to start 'at home', within the psychiatric profession, and continue through the mobilization of other branches of medicine to finally encompass the broader structure of society. Conceptual modifications and changes in the practice of psychiatry will be necessary if the fight against the stigma of mental disorders is given the priority that it deserves. International collaboration is likely to be useful in the development of relevant programs. The program against stigma and discrimination resulting from schizophrenia launched recently by the WPA aims to develop material for use in national programs and thus facilitate joint action and learning from each other.

References

1   Murray CJL, Lopez AD: The Global Burden of Disease. Boston, Harvard School of Public Health, 1996.
2   Sartorius N, deGirolamo G, Andrews G, German A, Eisenberg L (eds): Treatment of mental disorders: A review of effectiveness. Washington, American Psychiatric Press, 1993.
3   Sartorius N, Henderson AS: The neglect of prevention in psychiatry. Aust NZ J Psychiatry 1992; 26:550.
4   World Psychiatric Association: Fighting Stigma and Discrimination because of Schizophrenia. New York, World Psychiatric Association, 1998, vol 1 and 2.

Prof. Norman Sartorius, Clinique de psychiatrie 1, Département de psychiatrie,
Hôpitaux Universitaires de Genève, 2, chemin du Petit-Bel-Air, CH–1225 Chêne-Bourg

Guimón J, Fischer W, Sartorius N (eds): The Image of Madness. The Public Facing Mental
Illness and Psychiatric Treatment. Basel, Karger, 1999, pp 105–117

······················

Public Education for Community Care:
A New Approach

Geoffrey Wolff [a], *Soumitra Pathare* [b], *Tom Craig* [b], *Julian Leff* [a]

[a] Social, Genetic and Developmental Psychiatry Research Centre
  (Social Psychiatry Section), Institute of Psychiatry and
[b] Academic Department of Psychiatry, St Thomas's Hospital, UMDS, London, UK

Research by the Team for the Assessment of Psychiatric Services (TAPS)
has shown that only a minority of patients make social contact with ordinary
members of the public, including neighbours. With a view to improving the
social integration of these patients, it is important to find ways of increasing
their number of social contacts with ordinary members of the public and of
sustaining such relationships. Public attitudes clearly have a bearing on this.
Little is known, however, about the malleability of public attitudes or their
effect on patients' social integration. Only Cumming and Cumming [1] in
Canada and Gatherer and Reid [2] in Northamptonshire have evaluated a
public education campaign in the local community. Neither study was linked
to a specific facility and both studies found education to be ineffective.

To our knowledge, there has been no previous published evaluation of
an educational campaign linked to a specific facility. The question as to whether
such an intervention would be effective (or even harmful) therefore remains
unresolved. The aims of our educational programme were to increase knowledge about mental illness, to decrease wariness toward the mentally ill and to
promote the social integration of the patients.

Method

As a part of the closure of Tooting Bec Hospital, a large Victorian asylum in south
London, patients have been placed in staffed group houses in the local area. In 1993 such
facilities opened in two areas, Herne Hill (accommodating 9 patients) and Streatham Hill
(accommodating 14 patients). Both are urban areas, situated in the London borough of
Lambeth. Both areas have a high proportion of individuals in social classes I and II and a

significant Afro-Caribbean population. The underprivileged area score of Herne Hill is 31.15 and that of Streatham Hill area is 29.15. Details of the study are documented elsewhere [3–5] but are briefly described below.

Prior to the opening of these facilities, immediate neighbours living on the same street as these houses were interviewed. The interview consisted of questions dealing with: (1) demographic data, (2) knowledge of mental illness, (3) reactions towards the mentally ill, (4) knowledge of psychiatric hospital care, (5) knowledge of the shift to care in the community, (6) attitude to community care policy, and (7) opinion about the need for education [4].

A knowledge scale (maximum score = 10) was computed from the main knowledge variables [4] as follows: naming of mental illness – 4 points (1 point each for naming schizophrenia, manic depression, depression and anxiety); definition of mental handicap – 3 points (1 point each for including low IQ, from birth and a permanent state), giving an example of mental handicap – 1 point (for a correct type, e.g. Down's syndrome), distinguishing mental illness from mental handicap – 1 point (for at least one of normal versus low IQ, later onset versus from birth, or a process rather than a permanent state, knowing the mentally ill are not less intelligent – 1 point).

Subjects were administered the Community Attitudes to the Mentally Ill (CAMI) inventory [6]. This is a 40-statement inventory and the subjects were asked to rate each statement on a five-point scale (strongly agree, agree, neutral, disagree and strongly disagree). Subjects were also asked to complete a self-report inventory of questions about fear of and behavioural intentions toward the mentally ill constructed especially for this study. This was a 10-item questionnaire with a five-point response scale.

Three factors were extracted by factor analysis of the CAMI. These were labelled Fear & Exclusion, Social Control and Goodwill. Attitudinal scales (Fear & Exclusion, Social Control and Goodwill) were derived by calculating the mean value of the scores (on a 1 to 5 scale – with a higher value representing a greater tendency toward each respective attitude) for the items on the CAMI with loadings of greater than or equal to 0.50 on the respective factors. These are reported in a previous paper [4]. The derived scales were constructed for ease of computation and comparison and are distinguished from their respective raw factors by being represented in upper case lettering.

A behavioural intention score was derived by calculating the mean value of the scores (on a 1 to 5 scale – very likely, likely, neutral, unlikely, very unlikely – with a higher value representing a more positive intention) for the 3 behavioural intention items which correlated most highly (tau > 0.35) with Fear & Exclusion at the baseline survey [4]: 'Would you object to having mentally ill people living in your neighbourhood?', 'Would you be willing to work with somebody with a mental illness?', and 'Would you invite somebody into your home if you knew they suffered from mental illness?'.

The initial survey revealed that the majority of people expressed positive attitudes towards the mentally ill. There was an overwhelming majority who expressed attitudes of goodwill toward the mentally ill but a significant minority expressed fearful and socially controlling attitudes and people often expressed fears for the safety of children. There was an overwhelming desire for information about new community care facilities opening up. Neighbours were concerned that the patients should get adequate support and that they were not dangerous [3].

One of the areas (Streatham Hill) was chosen as the experimental area by tossing a coin. In this area, an educational campaign was conducted. The other area (Herne Hill) was designated the control area. The educational campaign comprised a primarily didactic component (an information pack containing a video and information sheets), a primarily social component (social events and social overtures from staff) and a mixed component (a formal reception and informal discussion sessions). Following the educational campaign, the survey was repeated in both areas (2 years after the initial survey and 1 year after the start of the educational campaign). In addition, supplementary questions were asked about people's perception of the staff and patients in the supported houses (see Appendix). The patients were assessed around the time of opening of the houses with the Present State Examination (PSE [7]), Social Behaviour Schedule (SBS [8]) and the Social Network Schedule (SNS [9]). The SBS and SNS were repeated 2 years after the opening of the houses in each area.

Analysis

Analysis was carried out using SPSS [10]. Analysis of differences between categorical variables between the two areas was carried out using the χ^2 test [using Fisher's exact test (FET) where necessary]. Tests of relationship between attitude scales and categorical variables were done using both independent and paired Student's t tests where the characteristic had two categories (e.g. contact with staff or patients) and using one-way ANOVA (with Bonferroni's correction) where there were more than two categories (e.g. interview status). Repeated measures ANOVA was used to determine the interaction between continuous variables (attitude scales and behavioural intentions scale) and categorical variables (such as area) over time. The effect sizes (the difference in means divided by the population standard deviation) were calculated for associations with Fear & Exclusion (SD = 0.67), Social Control (SD = 0.71) and Goodwill (SD = 0.51).

Results

There were 305 immediate neighbours of the two facilities. At baseline, 215 people (70% of the target population of 305) were interviewed (113/159 – 71% – in area 1 and 102/146 – 70% – in area 2). A further 90 (30%) were not interviewed, either because they refused (60/305 – 20%), could not be contacted (21/305 – 7%) or were unable to co-operate because of health problems or language differences (9/305 – 3%).

There were no differences in any of the sociodemographic variables between the two areas except that there were more people of higher social class in the experimental area and more Africans and Caribbeans in the control area. However, there were no overall differences in attitudes at baseline in the two areas (tables available from authors).

At the time of the second interviews, 109 (51%) of the original 215 respondents were interviewed. A further 66 (31%) had moved; 17 (8%) refused the repeat interview, and 23 (11%) could not be contacted, defaulted from their appointments or were unable to co-operate because of ill health (see table 1).

Negative attitudes at first interview were predictive of refusal to be reinterviewed. Effect sizes were as follows: Fear & Exclusion (1.23; p < 0.001), Social Control (1.22; p < 0.001) and Goodwill (0.66; p < 0.05). Subjects who

Table 1. Number of interviews: follow-up data

	Total (n = 215)		Control area (n = 113)		Experimental area (n = 102)	
	n	%	n	%	n	%
Interviewed	109	51	62	55	47	46
Moved	66	31	28	25	38	37
Refused	17	8	13	12	4	4
Defaulted	12	6	6	5	6	6
Not contacted	9	4	4	4	5	5
Unable	2	1	0	0	2	2

Difference between control and experimental area: $\chi^2 = 9.92$; d.f. = 5; non-significant.

moved or who were not interviewed for other reasons showed no difference from those who were interviewed in terms of the attitudinal factors (table available from authors). There were some missing data hence data on CAMI scales were only available on 98–100/109 respondents and Fear and Behavioural Intentions data were only available on 105/109 respondents.

Changes in Knowledge and Attitudes at Follow-Up

There was no significant difference between increase in knowledge in the two areas over time. However, there was a non-significant trend toward a greater increase in knowledge in the experimental area when only the neighbours who had participated in the educational campaign (i.e. those who had at least seen the information pack) were compared with those in the control area (see table 2).

In the experimental area, neighbours who took up the educational material showed an increase in knowledge compared to those who did not (see table 2). However, there was no direct relationship between having been educated and change in attitudes over time.

Overall Changes in Attitudes

There was an overall decrease in Fear & Exclusion (effect size 0.41) in the experimental area at follow-up compared to the control area (see table 3). There was no change in Social Control or Goodwill.

Overall Changes in Behavioural Intentions

There was an overall increase in respondents' behavioural intention scores (effect size 0.51) in the experimental area at follow-up but not in the control

Table 2. Knowledge scores at baseline and follow-up in the control area versus the experimental area who were and who were not educated

	Baseline	Follow-up
Control area (n = 62)	3.7 (2.4)	4.3 (2.5)
Experimental area		
Not educated (n = 16)	4.5 (2.3)	4.4 (2.1)
Educated (n = 31)	4.6 (2.7)	6.1 (2.4)

Values represent mean with the SD in parentheses. RMANOVA (Bonferroni's correction): group by knowledge: control vs. those educated – p = 0.06; experimental area (educated) vs. experimental area (not educated) – p < 0.05.

Table 3. Fear & Exclusion, Social Control and Goodwill at baseline and follow-up in the two areas

	Baseline	Follow-up
Fear & Exclusion[a]		
Control area (n = 55)	2.13 (0.73)	2.11 (0.74)
Experimental area (n = 43)	2.25 (0.75)	1.97 (0.60)
Social Control[b]		
Control area (n = 55)	2.17 (0.71)	2.20 (0.74)
Experimental area (n = 45)	2.16 (0.65)	2.08 (0.57)
Goodwill[c]		
Control area (n = 55)	4.34 (0.49)	4.35 (0.53)
Experimental area (n = 44)	4.32 (0.45)	4.27 (0.56)

Values represent mean with the SD in parentheses.
[a] RMANOVA area by Fear & Exclusion; p < 0.05.
[b] RMANOVA area by Social Control; non-significant.
[c] RMANOVA area by Goodwill; non-significant.

area (see table 4). This indicates increased reported acceptance of patients in the experimental area.

Neighbours' Contact with Staff and Patients

Neighbours in the experimental area were more likely to make contact with both staff [79% (37/47) vs. 19% (12/62); $\chi^2 = 38.09$; d.f. = 1; p < 0.001] and patients [94% (44/47) vs. 71% (44/62); $\chi^2 = 8.82$; d.f. = 1; p < 0.01]. This included

Table 4. Behavioural intention scores at baseline and follow-up in the control area versus the experimental area

	Baseline	Follow-up
Control area (n=60)	4.09 (0.84)	4.09 (0.80)
Experimental area (n=45)	3.86 (0.63)	4.19 (0.66)

Values represent mean with the SD in parentheses.
RMANOVA area by behavioural intentions; p<0.01.

Table 5. Fear & Exclusion at baseline and follow-up versus contact with staff and patients: experimental area

	Baseline	Follow-up	p
Contact with staff[a]			
No contact with staff (n=9)	2.08 (0.57)	2.07 (0.39)	NS
Contact with staff (n=34)	2.29 (0.79)	1.94 (0.65)	<0.001[c]
Contact with patients[b]			
No contact with patients (n=3)	1.91 (0.81)	2.21 (0.50)	NS
Contact with patients (n=40)	2.28 (0.75)	1.95 (0.61)	<0.001[c]

Values represent mean with the SD in parentheses.
[a] RMANOVA contact with staff by Fear & Exclusion: non-significant.
[b] RMANOVA contact with patients by Fear & Exclusion: p=0.05.
[c] Student's t test (paired).

all levels of contact from passing in the street to making friendships. They were more likely, for example, than those in the control area to attend a social event in one of the houses [21% (10/47) vs. 7% (4/62); $\chi^2=5.25$; d.f.=1; p<0.05].

It was neighbours who showed more Fear & Exclusion at baseline who tended to make contact with staff and patients. In the experimental area, there was an overall decrease in Fear & Exclusion over time in respondents who had contact with patients (effect size 0.49) compared with those who did not. There was also a decrease in Fear & Exclusion in respondents who had contact with staff but this did not reach significance when compared with the group who had no contact (see table 5). Given the small numbers in the group who did not make contact, this may well be a type II error. There was no change in Social Control or Goodwill.

Neighbours in the experimental area were more likely to know the names of staff [57% (27/47) vs. 7% (4/62); $\chi^2 = 34.16$; d.f = 1; p<0.001] or count them as friends [13% (6/47) vs. 0% (0/62); $\chi^2 = 8.38$; d.f. = 1; p<0.01]. They were also more likely to know the names of patients [28% (13/47) vs. 8% (5/62); $\chi^2 = 7.45$; d.f. = 1; p<0.01] and they were more likely to have had higher levels of social interaction such as visiting them [28% (13/47) vs. 8% (5/62)]; and inviting them in or counting them as friends [13% (6/47) vs. 0% (0/62); $\chi^2 = 17.72$; d.f. = 2; p<0.001].

All the respondents in the experimental area who made friends with patients (n=4) or invited them into their homes (n=2) found out about the supported houses because of this project. Neighbours in the experimental area were also less likely to report problems such as being shouted at in the street, being asked for money or being followed by patients [9% (4/47) vs. 45% (28/62); $\chi^2 = 17.32$; d.f. = 1; p<0.001].

Patients' Illness, Behaviour and Social Networks

Patients were considerably disabled but there were no significant differences between the two areas. PSE data were only available on 19 patients. Most (12/19) had an index of definition of 7 or 8. Mean total PSE score was 16.

SBS data were available on all patients. Most had problems with social behaviour (SBS item scores of 2 or more). Most had problems with personal hygiene [74% (17/23)] and underactivity [52% (12/23)]. Other common problems were lack of initiative in communication [26% (6/23)], incoherence in conversation [22% (5/23)], inability to make social contacts in an appropriate way [22% (5/23)], and problems with concentration [22% (5/23)]. There was no significant difference between change in social behaviour problems over time in the two areas.

Baseline SNS data were available on 15 of the 23 patients. Patients had a mean of 14 social contacts (SD=6.5). None of the patients had any contact with neighbours. There were no significant differences between the two areas in these measures.

At follow-up there were only 8 patients in the control area (1 had died and 1 was transferred back to hospital and a further patient admitted in her place) and 12 patients in the experimental area (1 had been transferred and 1 was in respite care). At follow-up, only 6 of the 8 patients in the control area and 8 of the 12 patients in the experimental area were willing or able to co-operate with questions about their social networks.

In the experimental area, at follow-up, most patients (5/8) reported having made contact (each contact at least monthly) with neighbours compared with none (0/6) in the control area ($\chi^2 = 5.8$, d.f. = 1; p<0.05 – FET). There was a mean of 2 (SD=2.0) contacts with neighbours per patient in the experimental area compared with 0 in the control area (p < 0.05). In all, there were 13 reported regular contacts with neighbours in the experimental area (4 monthly, 8 weekly and 1 daily). Two patients each reported that they considered three neighbours to be friends.

Discussion

Difficulties in Mounting the Campaign

It may be surprising to some that this piece of research met with major resistance. It was not granted ethical approval in other areas of London; probably because of fear of provoking a backlash against the facilities and because of concerns about confidentiality. It was, therefore, welcomed when the opportunity arose to conduct the study in West Lambeth.

The educational campaign was planned in consultation with staff from the supported houses in Streatham Hill. However, various problems arose. Some staff objected to the educational campaign in principle on the grounds of normalisation ideology; they were concerned that it might draw attention to the patients and that there was no reason to encourage their integration into the community as they were just the same as anybody else and they should not be labelled as mentally ill. These issues are not peculiar to this study. Marks [11] commented on the re-emergence of antipsychiatry in the non-medical professions that make up the major part of our community mental health services.

Others did not believe that neighbours were interested and did not feel it would have any beneficial effects for the patients. Practical considerations such as staffing levels often made it difficult for staff to find time to put into the project. These problems needed addressing at various stages as the project progressed. Thus time needed to be spent with staff providing explanations of the rationale of the study and on feedback about the very positive response from the neighbours.

These issues held back the progress of the educational campaign considerably, otherwise it would have been conducted much closer to the opening of the houses and would have been completed much faster. Indeed, neighbours clearly would have liked information around the time the houses opened or before, as rumours spread like Chinese whispers and they felt that there had been secrecy, surrounding the houses.

At baseline, an overwhelming number of respondents (91%) had expressed a desire for information [3]. However, only around a third (34/102) of the sample in the experimental area took up the offer of educational material.

The issue of confidentiality and privacy clearly arises in any undertaking of this nature hence the patients were asked and gave their consent for the campaign. Although neighbours would have liked patients to be in the video it was felt that this would be too intrusive.

Possible Confounding Factors

This was an opportunistic study with the experimenters having no control over the siting or structure of the services, or number or level of disability of the residents in the houses. It may be, therefore, that there were confounding characteristics in the facilities themselves or in the neighbours in the two areas. This possibility is explored below.

There were differences in the social class and ethnic mix of the neighbours in the two areas with more people of higher social class in the experimental area and more Africans and Caribbeans in the control area. These may affect willingness to take up educational opportunities and to complain but although people of higher social class have more favourable attitudes and Africans and Caribbeans have less favourable attitudes [4], there were no overall differences in attitudes at baseline in the two areas.

There were also differences in the supported houses in each area. In the experimental area there was a cluster of three houses and in the control area only one. This may have led to a higher profile in this area. However, there was no difference in the number of people who had heard comments about the houses from neighbours (22 in each area). There were differences, at follow-up, in the relative ratio of positive and negative comments people had heard, with over twice as many negative comments in the control area [68% (15/22) vs. 32% (7/22)] and over 3 times as many positive comments in the experimental area [36% (8/22) vs. 9% (2/22); $\chi^2 = 6.84$; d.f. $= 2$; p < 0.05].

There were more patients in the experimental area. This might explain why more neighbours had made contact with residents. However, one might also have expected more problems reported in this area whereas the reverse was the case with more problems being reported in the control area. There was no overall difference in SBS or SNS data in the patients in the two areas which might account for the differences found.

There may have been bias in the rating of the semistructured interview, but raters applied strict rating criteria and changes in attitude were reflected in the self-report questionnaires, therefore, this is unlikely to have been a major confounding influence. Finally, social desirability response set probably affected results in both areas equally. For these reasons, it seems unlikely that these confounding variables significantly influenced the results.

Outcome of the Attitude Survey

The results of the follow-up survey suggest that although the public education intervention may have, at best, only a modest effect on knowledge, it is associated with an improvement in overall attitudes and behaviour toward the mentally ill (with a decrease in fear and exclusion and increased levels of social contact) in the experimental area. This is consistent with the finding of Berkowitz et al. [12] who found that even small changes in knowledge following an educational programme for relatives of patients with schizophrenia were associated with important changes in attitude and behaviour toward patients.

However, the education campaign did not in itself lead directly to less fearful attitudes, whereas contact with patients did. It is likely, therefore, that the campaign exerted its effect on overall attitudes indirectly by encouraging contact with patients. Such contact may well exert its effect on attitudes, in part, by the reassurance such contact gives about the two main concerns of neighbours about new facilities in their area. These concerns are to do with wanting to know whether the patients are adequately supported and whether or not they are likely to be dangerous [3].

Patients' Assessments

The findings from the attitude survey are clearly supported by the patients' accounts, with several of the patients in the experimental area, but none in the control area, reporting having made contact and even friendships with neighbours. Indeed, 2 out of 8 of the patients in the experimental area interviewed at follow-up had made friendships with neighbours. To put this in context, about a third of all neighbours had reported at baseline interview that they had made friendships with other neighbours. Sadly, when asked about whether he had any contact with neighbours, one resident in the control area replied: 'Of course not, how can I see the neighbours, this is a psychiatric unit, not a private home'. Perhaps patients also need to be involved in discussion regarding their perception of their position in the community.

Suggestions

The intervention is fairly time-consuming but it can be taken at a slow pace and any effort expended has a knock-on effect as there is an indirect dissemination of information from neighbour to neighbour. This is important given that a significant number of neighbours were not directly reached by the campaign.

In order to make the maximum continuing impact with the minimum outlay in time and effort the following suggestions may be helpful. Firstly, it may be useful to target groups with the most negative attitudes. People with children in the household and Africans and Caribbeans, for example, are the groups which are more likely to object to the mentally ill in the community [4]. Secondly, repeating the reception for people who could not attend the first time and seeing neighbours together rather than individually may well allow the campaign to reach a greater proportion of the local population without taking up too much more time. Thirdly, it may be better to see neighbours in small groups as work has shown that it is easier to change attitudes in individuals formed in a group [13] and the changes are more permanent [14]. Fourthly, momentum in campaigns is of vital importance. The effect on attitudes of several interventions is greater than the sum of the effect of each [15]. In order to keep up momentum it is important to have an enthusiastic staff member who will continue the campaign and it may be useful to organise interested neighbours to become befrienders and to help with continuing liaison with neighbours both new and established.

Conclusions

These findings, although tentative, have important implications for the re-integration of psychiatric patients into the community. Fear of a backlash as experienced by Cumming and Cumming [1] or a hardening of attitudes by such an intervention are clearly not borne out by this study. The authors hope this may well pave the way to greater openness and involvement of local residents around new or existing facilities in the future and encourage others to explore similar ways of improving patients' social integration.

Clinical Implications
The public education intervention may be used to improve patients' social integration. The intervention helps to allay neighbours' fears. It is hoped that this work will lead to greater openness and public consultation around new and existing facilities.

Limitations
There could be uncontrolled variables mediating the differences in the two areas and patient numbers were small. The study needs replication. Staff reservations need to be overcome for the intervention to be successful. The intervention has little effect on neighbours' knowledge about mental illness.

Acknowledgements

We are grateful to Mr Greedharee, manager of the supported houses, for his efforts in liaising with the local community, and conducting informal discussion sessions with neighbours. Our thanks are also due to John Allinson for his production of the video, The Gatsby Charitable Foundation for its generous sponsoring of the video, and to those, including Catherine Gamble and Jane Rogers, who took part in the making of the video.

Appendix

Supplementary Questions Regarding People's Perception of Staff and Patients in the Supported Houses

What contact did they have with staff from the supported houses? Did they know the names of any of them? Would they count any of the staff as friends?

What contact did they have with residents from the supported houses? Did they know the names of any of them? What type of contact did they have [had no contact or saw them in street only/greeted them occasionally/had casual conversations with them/exchanged small favours/visited them (how many times?)/ invited them in/made friendships with any of them]? Had they had any problems with them?

Did the subject attend reception, see video, read information sheets, attend a social event at one of the houses (e.g. barbecue) or have any other contact?

Had other people commented about the supported houses or about the patients/residents? If yes: What did they say? (specify).

What was their opinion about the supported houses/residents? Had any other people commented about the information/educational campaign? If yes: What did they say? (specify).

What was the respondent's/your opinion about the information/educational campaign?

References

1 Cumming E, Cumming J: Closed Ranks – An Experiment in Mental Health Education. Cambridge, Harvard University Press, 1957.
2 Gatherer A, Reid JJA: Public Attitudes and Mental Health Education. Northamptonshire Mental Health Project, 1963.
3 Wolff G, Pathare S, Craig T, Leff J: Who's in the lions' den? The community's perception of community care for the mentally ill. Psychiatr Bull 1996;20:68–71.
4 Wolff G, Pathare S, Craig T, Leff J: Community attitudes to mental illness. Br J Psychiatry 1996; 168:183–190.
5 Wolff G, Pathare S, Craig T, Leff J: Community knowledge of mental illness and reaction to mentally ill people. Br J Psychiatry 1996;168:191–198.
6 Taylor MS, Dear MJ: Scaling community attitudes toward the mentally ill. Schizophr Bull 1981;7: 225–240.
7 Wing JK, Cooper JE, Sartorius N: Measurement and Classification of Psychiatric Symptoms. Cambridge, Cambridge University Press, 1974.
8 Wykes T, Sturt E: The measurement of social behaviour in psychiatric patients: An assessment of the reliability and validity of the SBS schedule. Br J Psychiatry 1986;148:1–11.
9 Dunn M, O'Driscoll C, Dayson D, Wills W, Leff J: The TAPS Project. 4. An observational study of the social life of long-stay patients. Br J Psychiatry 1990;157:842–848.
10 Norusis MJ: SPSS/PC+ V2.0 Base Manual. Chicago, SPSS, 1988.
11 Marks J: The re-emergence of antipsychiatry. Hosp Update 1994;20:187–190.

12   Berkowitz R, Shavit N, Leff JP: Educating relatives of schizophrenic patients. Soc Psychiatry Psychi-
      atr Epidemiol 1990;25:216–220.
13   Lewin K: Group decision and social change; in Swanston G, Newcomb T, Hartley E (eds): Readings
      in Social Psychology. New York, Holt, 1952.
14   Olmsted MS: The Small Group. New York, Random House, 1959.
15   Allport GW: The Nature of Prejudice. New York, Addison-Wesley, 1954.

Dr. Geoffrey Wolff, MRC Social, Genetic and Developmental Psychiatry Research Centre
(Social Psychiatry Section), Institute of Psychiatry,
DeCrespigny Park, Denmark Hill, London SE5 8AF (UK)
Tel. +44 0113 275 5734

Guimón J, Fischer W, Sartorius N (eds): The Image of Madness. The Public Facing Mental Illness and Psychiatric Treatment. Basel, Karger, 1999, pp 118–128

....

Combatting the Alienation Experienced by People with Mental Illness

Richard Warner

Mental Health Center of Boulder County, Boulder, Colo., USA

Alienation is a serious problem – serious enough that, in 1972, the US Senate commissioned research into the effects of alienation in the workplace [1]. It is a central concern also, for radical psychiatrist, R.D. Laing. 'Alienation goes to the roots', he wrote, '... this realization unites men as diverse as Marx, Kierkegaard, Nietzsche, Freud, Heidegger, Tillich and Sartre' [2, p. 12]. The Senate was concerned about falling productivity, Laing about the estrangement of humanity 'from its authentic possibilities'. Others worry about anomie and crime among inner-city youth and others still about the effect of alienation upon the physical and mental health of a broad stratum of society [3]. In this paper, I shall be concerned with the impact of alienation on the seriously mentally ill, and the extent to which it stands in the way of recovery from psychosis. I shall describe some ways in which we may tackle this problem of alienation by means of normalizing domestic treatment settings and empowering consumer-run programs.

The mentally ill may be the most alienated people in our society. They confront the elements of alienation – meaninglessness, powerlessness, normlessness and estrangement from society and work – in their most extreme forms.

Meaninglessness

In discussing the theme of *Death of a Salesman*, Arthur Miller referred to '... a need greater than hunger, or sex, or thirst, the need to leave a thumbprint somewhere on the world' – in essence, the need to make some meaning of one's existence.

Meaning and meaninglessness are core existential concerns which confront us all [4]. Maddi [5] and others [4] describe an existential neurosis presenting as chronic meaninglessness, aimlessness and apathy coupled with boredom, depression and blunted affect. Those who work with people with long-standing mental illness will recognize these features as common among their clients. What puts them so much at risk?

Most of the mentally ill people in the community have little or nothing to do. In a study which my colleagues and I conducted in Boulder, Colo., for example, we found that half of the mentally ill in the community had no more than 1 hour of structured activity each day [6]. Lacking a useful social role, many people with mental illness face lives of profound purposelessness. Psychotic patients, in fact, score lower than any other group on the Purpose-in-Life Test [7].

In one recent study, when people in community treatment for psychosis were interviewed about their lives, their principal complaints were of boredom and (among the men) unemployment – both rated as much more problematic than psychotic symptoms [8].

Many professionals suspect that the high prevalence of drug and alcohol abuse among the mentally ill – 30–40% of most samples [9, 10] – is in part a consequence of the empty lives which many patients lead. In a study of substance use among the mentally ill in Boulder, we found that those with the fewest planned activities were the heaviest marijuana users, giving 'boredom' as the primary reason for drug use.

Depression, another feature of the existential neurosis, is also common in schizophrenia. The Iowa record linkage study [11] reveals that completed suicide is 30 times the general population rate in schizophrenic men and 60 times the expected rate in schizophrenic women – a higher rate even than in affective disorder. It is clear that many, perhaps most, of the chronically mentally ill in the community display the full range of features of the existential neurosis.

Decades ago, when we were shifting the locus of care from the hospital to the community, we found ways to combat what we called at that time the institutional neurosis – the posturing, the restless pacing, incontinence and unpredictable violence which were bred by the restrictions, regimentation and emptiness of hospital life. Humanizing the hospital wards and establishing 'therapeutic communities', which changed the power relationships between staff and patients and involved patients in ward management, led to a reversal of this institutionally ingrained behavior [12, 13]. It now appears that we have traded the earlier *institutional* neurosis for a new *existential* neurosis which may similarly stand in the way of recovery from the original psychotic illness. We may find, however, that the same active ingredients which proved successful in reversing the institutional syndrome – normalizing the environment and engaging the patient in his or her own treatment – will also prove effective in relieving the effect of the existential neurosis.

Powerlessness

Meaninglessness and the associated elements of the existential neurosis are only some of the components of the alienation which threatens the mentally ill. It is also true to say that the mentally ill are some of the most powerless people in our society. One of the triumphs of modern community treatment of the mentally ill has been to demonstrate that intensive outpatient case management programs can virtually eliminate relapse and admission to hospital [14]. This is good news for people with schizophrenia and manic-depressive illness, practically all of whom say that they would much rather be out of hospital than in [15].

Effective relapse prevention programs, however, tend to be quite controlling. In fact, in those states where the mental illness statute allows it, these programs may make considerable use of outpatient certification for involuntary treatment.

A piece of research which we conducted at our agency in Boulder leads me to be particularly worried about the issue of control. Most professionals would argue that a person with mental illness needs to understand that he or she is mentally ill in order to benefit from treatment. Our study of seriously mentally ill people living in the community [16], however, indicates that accepting the label of mental illness, by itself, is not associated with improved functioning: something more is needed. An internal locus of control – a sense of mastery over life – is essential if someone with a psychosis is to get any benefit from the knowledge that he or she suffers from a mental illness.

It also emerged from our study, though, that one of the consequences of accepting that one is mentally ill is a loss of the sense of self-mastery and self-esteem. In accepting the label, the person also takes on the stigma and western stereotype of the degraded, incompetent mental patient. This is the Catch-22 of being mentally ill in Western society – that one loses the very psychological strength which is necessary for recovery in the process of gaining knowledge and insight. We concluded, from our research, that it is as important for our patients to develop a sense of self-mastery as it is for them to accept the fact that they are ill. Conventional treatment programs, however, with their element of control, cannot help much in developing the lost sense of mastery. The question for the therapist and patient is how to offset the controlling effects of relapse prevention. One solution, I suggest, is to empower the patient through involvement in consumer-run programs, and I will discuss some of these ventures in detail below.

Normlessness

The tendency for some mentally ill people to neglect certain codes of conduct can be a source of frustration to the therapist and others and may lead to the patient being labeled as having a personality disorder in addition to his or her psychosis. Why does this person steal? Why does that one seem to care so little for the effect his behavior has on others? If we reframe the behavior, in some cases, as being the product of anomie or normlessness arising from the patient's alienated state and from a damaged sense of belonging, we may find different ways to approach it. An attempt to engage the individual in a supportive but confrontative social group may be more productive than a punitive response. The use of the therapeutic community approach for the treatment of prisoners, drug addicts and character disorders is based, to an extent, upon this premise [12, 13].

Social Estrangement

The mentally ill are no longer so estranged from humankind that they are considered, as they were before the 17th century Age of Reason, as bestial. They continue, however, to be the most stigmatized group in our society. Their status is lower than that of ex-convicts or the mentally retarded [17]. The label of mental illness itself may produce adverse effects. A study of attitudes of residents of a small New England town shows that a normal person of an 'ideal type' who is described as having been in mental hospital is socially rejected to a much greater extent than is a schizophrenic who seeks no help or who instead consults a clergyman [18]. Stigma may have a crippling impact. Strauss and Carpenter ask:

'Who can doubt the devastating impact on a fragile person of perceiving that the entire social milieu regards him (wittingly or not) as subhuman, incurable, unmotivated, or incompetent to pursue ordinary expectations ...? Can we doubt that a deteriorating course of disorder is fostered when fundamental roles are changed by social stigma and employment opportunities become limited?' [19, p. 128]

Work Estrangement

We live in a society in which economists consider *full* employment to be 4–5% *un*employment. Those who are marginally productive are not likely to find work and keep it. Most of the mentally ill in the community are completely divorced from productive activity, and these unemployed patients are perhaps the most alienated. The effects on the patient's illness may be substantial. Some of the emotional reactions associated with long-term unemployment are so similar to the negative symptoms and secondary effects of schizophrenia they are all but indistinguishable: they include anxiety, depression, apathy, irritability, negativity, dependency, emotional withdrawal, isolation, loneliness, low self-esteem, loss of identity and loss of a sense of time [20]. I do not mean to suggest that the negative symptoms of schizophrenia are necessarily *caused* by unemployment but that enforced idleness *worsens* these features of the illness and that we should not look for improvement in them until we have successfully tackled the patient's alienation.

Unfortunately, those who are in work may not be much better off. The jobs available to the marginally productive mentally ill are often the most undesirable and alienating – temporary, tedious and unrewarding positions in the secondary labor force, such as washing dishes. Economic considerations may discourage mentally disabled people from seeking even these low-paid jobs. A survey of mentally ill people in the Boulder community which I conducted with economic development specialist and psychiatrist Paul Polak reveals that, if patients take a job, they need to earn $5 an hour plus health insurance to offset the loss of social security, Medicaid and other entitlements. Anything less does not make economic sense. Since most available jobs pay minimum wage (recently raised to $4.25 an hour) and offer no benefits such as health insurance, it is generally not smart to work.

Combatting Alienation

I have argued the case in some detail, elsewhere [21], that labor market conditions have a major effect in shaping social responses to the mentally ill, psychiatric treatment approaches and outcome from schizophrenia. The strikingly superior outcome from schizophrenia in Third World villages, for example, may be, in part, a consequence of the easy return of the recovering psychotic person to a productive role in village life. The post-World-War-II social psychiatry revolution in northern Europe, I submit, was stimulated by an acute labor shortage, and the high success rates achieved by moral treatment in early 19th century American mental hospitals may well have been attributable, in part, to the demand for labor in the new republic.

Moral treatment and the post-World-War-II therapeutic community approach were similar in many ways. The basic principles of moral treatment included the avoidance of coercion and the development, instead, of individual self-control (or moral restraint). Treatment settings were generally small and homelike and patients were encouraged to participate in work and social activities in an effort to create a normalizing environment which would promote self-control and the maintenance of social skills and help integrate the person back into the community as early as possible [22].

I suggest that when society has an urgent need to employ the labor of its more marginally productive members, psychiatry swings into action with highly effective rehabilitative techniques which are capable of producing much better outcome in schizophrenia. These methods, common to moral treatment and to the therapeutic community approach, are *humanizing* and *normalizing* techniques which *empower* the patient by *engaging him or her in treatment*. They have the effect of reducing the patient's alienation and assisting his or her reintegration into a productive relationship with society. These minimal-restraint approaches emphasize self-control and use small, comfortable (and, where possible, domestic) environments in which the patient takes an operational role. Patients are respected as people, and return to their normal lives in the community as soon as possible.

We now live in a society with a high rate of unemployment, and the possibilities of returning mentally ill people to a productive role are strictly limited. Despite these limitations, however, I believe that we can use some of the active ingredients of moral treatment and the therapeutic community to attack the problem of alienation and to improve the functioning and quality of life of mentally ill people in the community. I shall give some examples of how this is now being done successfully.

Domestic Alternatives to the Hospital

Psychiatric treatment, by labeling people as abnormal, removing them to institutions and, sometimes, using coercion, is inherently antinormalizing. Clinical programs can be designed, however, so that this tendency is minimized, especially if we create alternatives to the psychiatric hospital – the most coercive and socially destructive component of the treatment system [23].

Cedar House is a large house on a busy residential street in Boulder, Colo. [24]. Staffed, as one would staff an acute psychiatric hospital ward, with nurses, a psychiatrist and mental health workers, it functions as an alternative to psychiatric hospital for the acutely disturbed patients of the county mental health center. Like a hospital, it offers all the usual diagnostic and treatment services (except electroconvulsive therapy). Routine medical evaluations are performed on premises: patients requiring advanced medical and neurological investigation are referred to local physicians and hospital departments. Unlike a hospital, it is homelike, unlocked and noncoercive, and it costs less than a quarter as much as private hospital treatment.

As far as possible, Cedar House has the appearance of a middle-class home, not a hospital. Pets share the comfortable furniture with the residents and, on winter nights, a fire burns in the hearth. Staff and patients interact casually and share household duties. Residents come and go fairly freely (some attend work while in treatment), when they have negotiated passes with the therapist. Staff must encourage patients to comply willingly with treatment and house rules: no one can be strapped down, locked in or medicated by force. Many patients, nevertheless, are treated involuntarily at Cedar House under the provisions of the state mental illness statute; they accept the restrictions because the alternative is hospital treatment, which virtually none prefer.

The people who cannot be treated in the house are those who are violent, threatening or who repeatedly walk away. In practice, just about everybody with a psychotic depression, most people with an acute episode of schizophrenia and many people with mania can be treated in the facility. Cedar House has not entirely replaced locked hospital care, but it provides nearly two thirds of all the inpatient treatment for the mental health center's clients, and could provide an even greater proportion if more beds of this type were available.

During the 1970s and 1980s, Paul Polak and his associates at Southwest Denver Mental Health Center in Colorado established and operated a revolutionary system of family sponsor homes for the care of acutely disturbed psychiatric patients [25]. This program consisted of a number of private homes where patients were helped through their crises by carefully screened and selected families. Mobile teams of psychiatrists, nurses and other professionals provided treatment to the patients placed in the sponsor homes: rapid tranquilization was sometimes used in the management of acutely psychotic patients. The program proved to be suitable for the large majority of the agency's acute admissions and helped reduce the daily use of hospital beds to 1 per 100,000 of the catchment area population.

A network of family crisis homes based on the Southwest Denver model is currently in operation in Madison, Wisc. [26]. A dozen family homes provide care to a wide variety of people in crisis most of whom would otherwise be in hospital; nearly three quarters of these clients suffer from acute psychotic illness and others are acutely suicidal. Nearly half of the patients entering the program are admitted from the community as an alternative to hospital care; the remainder are in transition out of the hospital or are people with social crises. Violence by people admitted to crisis homes is almost never a problem. This is partly because of careful selection of appropriate clients and partly because clients feel privileged to be invited into another person's home – they try to behave with the courtesy of house guests.

Work

One of the principal ways in which people maintain their sense of worth and mastery is through work. To this end, some European countries have been successful in establishing businesses which provide integrated work environments for a large proportion of the mentally ill. These include 'social firms' in Germany [27] and – the most empowering model – worker cooperatives in Italy and Switzerland [28]. In Trieste and Pordenone in northeastern Italy, the consortia of cooperative businesses employ a mixed workforce of roughly equal numbers of mentally disabled and healthy workers in manufacturing and service enterprises. The enterprises include (in Trieste) a hotel, a restaurant, and a building renovation company, and (in Pordenone) office cleaning, collecting money from public telephones, and home help for the disabled. The consortia are large: the production of the Trieste consortium totaled $5 million in 1994, and in Pordenone, $7.5 million.

The significance of the European social firm is that it offers a bridge between the sheltered workshop, on the one hand, and supported employment in the competitive workforce, on the other. It expands the range of vocational options by creating employment that allows accommodation for fluctuating levels of performance in a nonsegregated working environment and opens the door for more people with mental illness to gain meaning and empowerment through work.

Consumer-Run Programs

In recent years, in the USA and elsewhere, consumers of mental health services have become increasingly involved in running their own programs. Consumer organizations have set up cooperative housing projects, drop-in centers, support group speaker's bureaus, telephone hot lines and a variety of other services.

A program developed by Russ Porter and his associates [29] at the Regional Assessment and Training Center (RATC) in Denver, Colo., is a good example of consumer involvement. In the Consumer Case Management Aide Training Program, people who have suffered from serious mental illness are trained, through 6 weeks of classroom education and several months of on-the-job training, to work with other mentally ill people. Graduates earn 21 hours of college credit and are hired, at standard rates of pay, as case management aides at community mental health centers in Colorado. They provide a number of services to their clients including applying for welfare entitlements, finding housing, and teaching living skills. After 10 years of program operation, more than a hundred consumer mental health workers have been employed throughout the service system, providing models for patients and staff alike of successful recovery from mental illness. Two thirds of the trainees continue to be successfully employed in the mental health system 2 years after graduation. The program has been so well received that RATC is now training consumers for other mental health staff positions, such as residential care workers and job coaches for clients in supported employment.

'The Heights' is a cooperative housing program in north Manhattan, in New York City, which integrates mentally ill and mentally healthy residents and employs the residents in the operation of the apartment building. Management responsibilities in this cooperative, which was established by Columbia University Community Services, the mental health agency for the area, are shared between an independent nonprofit housing corporation, which acts as landlord, the residents and the mental health team. Representatives of each of these three bodies form a council which screens and selects new residents and ensures that one third of the rooms are allocated to people with serious mental illness. The committee also appoints residents to paid positions, such as doorman, in the cooperative.

Patients who are admitted to the locked psychiatric ward of San Francisco General Hospital are provided with a peer counselor – someone who also suffers from mental illness and has had inpatient treatment. The peer counselor's job is to humanize the hospital environment by offering advice and support which are completely distinct from the professional hospital treatment. (Only in unusual circumstances does the peer counselor talk to the staff about information gathered from the patient.) The volunteer peer counselors are trained and supervised by Carol Patterson, a social worker who is herself a consumer.

One consumer action group has opened its own psychiatric clinic. The Capitol Hill Action and Recreation Group (CHARG), in Denver, is a coalition of consumers and professionals which has established a consumer-run drop-in center and a full-scale psychiatric clinic for the treatment of severely ill people. The clinic is directly accountable to an elected consumer board and to a second board comprised of professionals and other interested people. All matters of clinic policy require the consent of the consumer board. CHARG also provides consumer advocates for patients at the local state hospital, in boarding homes and in other locations. The advocates visit the hospital wards, attend treatment planning meetings and accompany clients to court hearings: among other services, they help clients find apartments, apply for public assistance, appeal adverse Social Security rulings and contest involuntary treatment certifications.

The consumer movement is gathering momentum in all parts of the world. In the US, two organizations, the National Mental Health Consumer Association and the National Alliance of Mental Patients vie for membership, sponsor national conferences, send speakers to professional meetings, combat stigma through media presentations and lobby for political objectives. Consumers are appointed to the governing boards of many mental health centers, and state regulations in California require that the boards of residential facilities include consumer members. Utah has a statewide network of 17 local consumer organizations. One operates a cafe and another has developed a drop-in center and a housing cooperative with a half-a-million dollar annual budget. The statewide organization, U-Can-Du, employs a staff of three consumers, holds an annual state consumer conference and is involved in system advocacy, providing input into the state mental health planning process.

Many observers would argue that one of the most important developments in US psychiatry in the past two decades has been the growth of organizations of relatives of people with serious mental illness. The National Alliance for the Mentally Ill has lobbied for improvements in services for people with mental illness, influencing decisions to direct public mental health funding to the most seriously disturbed and to focus research efforts on schizophrenia. Media reports of the mentally ill have changed in response to a drive by the Alliance to reduce stigma and to establish a new openness about psychiatric illness.

Many are hopeful that the next decade will see an equivalent growth in the organization of *direct* or *primary* consumers of mental health services. This would help to balance the paternalism and control, which are unavoidable elements of relapse prevention programs, with the empowerment offered by consumer-run services. Engagement in purposeful activity is one of the most effective solutions to the existential neurosis. Using some ingredients of the therapeutic community approach which helped us tackle the institutional syndrome in the postwar decades – patient participation in their own treatment and control over their environment – coupled with the normalizing effect of using small, domestic treatment settings may enable us to reduce the alienation which hampers recovery from mental illness.

References

1   US Senate Bill 3916, 1972.
2   Laing RD: The Politics of Experience. Baltimore, Penguin, 1967.
3   Jahoda M, Rush H: Work, Employment and Unemployment, University of Sussex Science Policy Research Unit Occasional Paper. Brighton, University of Sussex, 1980, No 12.
4   Yalom ID: Existential Psychotherapy. New York, Basic Books, 1980.
5   Maddi S: The existential neurosis. J Abnorm Psychol 1981;72:311–325.
6   Warner R, Taylor D, Wright J, Sloat A, Springett G, Arnold S, Weinberg H: Substance use among the mentally ill: Prevalence reasons for use and effects on illness. Am J Orthopsychiatry 1994;64: 30–39.

7   Robinson JP, Shaver PR: Measures of Social Psychological Attitudes. Ann Arbor, Institute for Social Research, 1969.
8   Fromkin KR: Gender Differences among Chronic Schizophrenics in the Perceived Helpfulness of Community-Based Treatment Programs; doctoral dissertation, University of Colorado, 1985.
9   Safer DJ: Substance abuse by young adult chronic patients. Hosp Community Psychiatr 1985;38: 853–858.
10 Atkinson RM: Importance of alcohol and drug abuse in psychiatric emergencies. Calif Med 1973; 118:1–4.
11 Black DW, Warrack G, Winokur G: The Iowa record-linkage study. I. Suicides and accidental deaths among psychiatric patients. Arch Gen Psychiatry 1985;42:71–75.
12 Jones M: Social Psychiatry in Practice: The Idea of the Therapeutic Community. Baltimore, Penguin, 1968.
13 Clark DH: Social Therapy in Psychiatry. Baltimore, Penguin, 1974.
14 Stein LI, Test MA: Alternative to mental hospital treatment. I. Conceptual model, treatment program, and clinical evaluation. Arch Gen Psychiatry 1980;37:392–397.
15 Warner R, Huxley P: Psychopathology and quality of life among mentally ill patients in the community: British and US samples compared. Br J Psychiatry 1993;163:505–509.
16 Warner R, Taylor D, Powers M, Hyman J: Acceptance of the mental illness label by psychotic patients: Effects on functioning. Am J Orthopsychiatry 1989;59:398–409.
17 Tringo RL: The hierarchy of preference towards disability groups. J Spec Educ 1970;4:295–306.
18 Phillips DL: Public identification and acceptance of the mentally ill. Am J Public Health 1966;56: 755–763.
19 Strauss JS, Carpenter WT: Schizophrenia. New York, Plenum, 1981.
20 Eisenberg P, Lazarsfeld PF: The psychological effects of unemployment. Psychol Bull 1938;35: 358–390.
21 Warner R: Recovery from Schizophrenia: Psychiatry and Political Economy. London, Routledge & Kegan Paul, 1985.
22 Jones K: A History of Mental Health Services. London, Routledge & Kegan Paul, 1972.
23 Warner R: Alternatives to Hospital for Acute Psychiatric Treatment. Washington, American Psychiatric Press, 1995.
24 Warner R, Wollesen C: Cedar House: A non-coercive hospital alternative in Boulder, Colorado; in Warner R (ed): Alternatives to Hospital for Acute Psychiatric Treatment. Washington, American Psychiatric Press, 1995.
25 Polak PR, Kirby MW, Deitchman WS: Treating acutely ill psychotic patients in private homes; in Warner R (ed): Alternatives to Hospital for Acute Psychiatric Treatment. Washington, American Psychiatric Press, 1995.
26 Bennett R: The Crisis Home Program of Dane County; in Warner R (ed): Alternatives to Hospital for Acute Psychiatric Treatment. Washington, American Psychiatric Press, 1995.
27 Stastny P, Gelman R, Mayo H: The German experience with employing people in 'social firms' with psychiatric disabilities. IDEAS Portfolio IV, 4–5. New York, Rehabilitation International, 1992.
28 Polak P, Warner R: The economic life of seriously mentally ill people in the community. Psychiatr Serv 1996, 47:270–274.
29 Sherman PS, Porter MA: Mental health consumers as case management aides. Hosp Community Psychiatr 1991;42:494–498.

Prof. R. Warner, Mental Health Center of Boulder County,
1333 Iris Avenue, Boulder, CO 80304 (USA)
Tel. +1 303 443 8500, Fax +1 303 449 6029

Guimón J, Fischer W, Sartorius N (eds): The Image of Madness. The Public Facing Mental Illness and Psychiatric Treatment. Basel, Karger, 1999, pp 129–137

....

Group Therapy and Attitudinal Changes to Mental Illness in Medical Students

L. Yllá, A. González-Pinto

University of the Basque Country, Lejona, Spain

Group psychotherapy in all its various modalities has the common object of fostering the introspection, interior development and overall maturation of the subject with a view to facilitating behavioral changes and the ability to resolve conflicts. To this end emotional exchanges within a group context are of fundamental importance.

One of the best ways of studying group dynamics and the efficiency of group processes in achieving symptomatic and attitudinal changes in group members is to study training and sensitization groups.

In recent years, growing interest in the changes brought about in sensitization groups has been manifest, although there are still relatively few studies dealing with the subject, with the exception of the now classical studies of Lieberman et al. [1] and Yalom [2], and the more recent studies of Oppenheimer [3], Mackenzie [4, 5], Guimón et al. [6, 7], and González-Pinto et al. [8, 9]. These studies have provided evidence of certain clinical modifications in treated patients as well as changes in levels of personal satisfaction in different personality traits and in social adjustment.

The clinical efficacy of group psychotherapy has been demonstrated in studies which include meta-analysis of previously obtained results from level IV and V studies [10, 11]. Various changes in the symptomatology of post-graduate and undergraduate students, who had participated in different group experiments, have already been reported by our research team [7, 12–15].

The evaluation of attitudinal changes brought about by the experience of group therapy has required the use of certain 'measurement' techniques. Subjective questionnaires, autoapplied by group members, and centered upon the expectations of the group and the achievements of the process have been used by Janosik [16]. Mackenzie and Dies [17] elaborated and applied a more complex protocol, known as 'The CORE Battery'. We have applied this measurement technique in some of our own previous studies [7, 8].

Our research team has been interested in the changes of certain attitudes towards mental illness brought about in medical students and professionals from the same field [12–14, 18]. The attitude of the general public towards mental illness has been studied by Yllá et al. [12, 13, 19, 20] using a version of the OMI protocol (Opinions towards Mental Illness) devised by Cohen and Struening [21, 22] and adapted by Yllá [19] and Ozámiz [23].

Among different studies about 'attitudes towards psychiatry', the one elaborated in 1980 by the Avon Committee of General Practitioners in Great Britain [24] stands out. This work made evident a certain ignorance about mental illness and its therapeutic approach and a negative attitude towards nonpharmacological therapeutic methods (psychotherapies) and the widespread acceptance of the notion that the treatment of people with emotional problems was a general practitioner's task.

A change of attitude towards mental illness is an essential part of the educational process, not only of the future psychiatrists but also of general practitioners, especially since they play an important role for patients with mental pathology.

Several studies carried out in general hospitals by Ayuso [25], Ayuso and Calvé [26] and Díez Manrique et al. [27], also show that a rejection of mental illness is widespread in the medical professions. In recent years, many authors have been attempting to modify negative attitudes in the field of mental health. In particular, modifications in attitudes towards psychodrugs and their use have been investigated by Lesser et al. [28], Payn [29], and Eguiluz [30].

In our environment a new study in a general hospital was carried out by García Ruiz et al. [18] with the purpose of assessing the medical staff's attitude towards the psychiatry service of the hospital, mental illness, and psychiatry in general. In contrast to the findings obtained in previous years, attitudes with regard to psychiatry and mental illness were found to be generally more positive and at the same time more critical. The authors of this work postulated that the aforementioned change could be related to a better integration of psychiatry into clinical practice, and suggested that the way to change stereotypes is through feedback, that is bringing into the system the results obtained from its functioning [19].

Knowledge of and proximity to the mentally sick subjects have been reported as inducing more favorable attitudes to mental illness [31–33]. Clarke [34] and Zwiebel [35] report that psychiatric training which includes approaching psychiatric patients in addition to cognitive activities is effective in modifying attitudes to mental illness. Moreover, Balint [36], among other authors, pointed out that good psychological information and formation of the health staff results in a better physician-patient relationship.

Attitudes can also be modified by psychotherapy, in which a greater understanding of the deep motivations at the root of such attitudes may alter the affective components as well as the cognitive elements of such attitudes.

The aim of the present study is to analyze whether any change in attitudes towards the mentally sick and towards psychiatric illness was brought about in medical students from the University of the Basque Country, by means of group psychotherapy sensitization sessions and/or group sessions of approach to the psychiatric patient from the study of psychiatric cases.

Materials and Methods

This study was carried out at the Medical School of the University of the Basque Country. Forty-eight second-year medical students, who agreed to participate voluntarily in a group experience, were randomly assigned to four groups – two of them were theoretical formative groups (of approach to the mental illness in the sense described above) and two experiential groups (of sensitization to psychodynamic process). All students filled in the OMI-R questionnaire both before and after the group training experience.

Each of the experiental groups initially consisted of 12 students. The total number of subjects in these groups was 24. Three students from these groups left. These 'psychoanalytic' groups (in Foulkes' [37] sense of the word) underwent a sensitization process. They were conducted by two teachers experienced in group analysis. We call it sensitization process because we cannot consider the groups as traditional psychotherapy groups given the conditions under which they were assembled (short time, lack of periodicity between sessions) due to the academic calendar.

The two theoretical groups were likewise made up of 24 students, 12 persons each, but 5 left. The teachers in these groups tried to develop an approach which would favor the mentally ill and mental illness through the display of clinical case histories and by group discussion about the individual cases.

The sessions for both theoretical and experiential groups were similar in duration (60 min), frequency and location (Medical Psychology Unit) and they took place between the months of October and April because of the academic calendar.

Measurement Techniques

In order to measure attitudes towards mental illness we used the OMI-R, a Spanish adaptation [19, 23] of the Cohen and Struening questionnaire OMI. The questionnaire is made up of 60 items which cover the following five dimensions: authoritarianism, benevolence, interpersonal etiology, restrictivity and negativism. Research with this questionnaire has been done in recent years to evaluate the general population's [38], physicians' and students' attitude toward mental illness [39, 40] and the influence of psychiatric courses on students' attitudes toward mental disease [41].

Table 1. Changes in attitudinal components toward mental illness in medical students

Attitudinal components	Theoretical group (n = 19)	Experiential group (n = 21)
Authoritarianism		
Before	80.6 (2.2)	83.6 (1.8)
After	84.2 (2.4)*	85.2 (2.0)
Interpersonal etiology		
Before	32.8 (1.0)	32.9 (1.2)
After	31.9 (0.7)	32.3 (1.3)
Benevolence		
Before	14.9 (0.6)	15.5 (0.6)
After	15.3 (0.7)	15.0 (0.6)
Restrictivity		
Before	20.3 (0.4)	20.3 (0.4)
After	20.5 (0.4)	20.3 (0.5)
Negativism		
Before	49.3 (1.0)	46.9 (0.7)
After	47.9 (1.0)	47.5 (0.8)

Values represent mean with the SD in parentheses. $*p < 0.05$.

Statistical Methods

Before-after differences within groups were assessed by paired t tests whereas differences between groups were tested by covariance analysis. Graphical exploratory analysis (box and density plots) were also performed to inspect the score distributions. All the analyses were performed with SYSTAT [42].

Results

As can be seen in table 1, the only dimension which increases is authoritarianism. When each group is considered separately, it can be seen that only in the theoretical groups the difference is significant (t value = 2.25 on 18 d.f.; p = 0.038).

Authoritarianism is the fundamental component of the attitude towards mental illness as is demonstrated by factorial analysis of the 60 items of the OMI-R scale. In a previous study, it accounted for 54.28% of the variance [19,23]. This factor refers to the necessity of isolation and custody of the

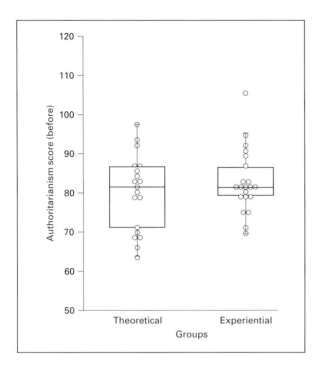

Fig. 1. Authoritarianism (before) according to the two groups.

mentally sick and shows a pessimistic position in relation to the possibility of healing.

The content of the authoritarian items of the OMI-R scale refers to: (1) the necessity of isolation of mentally ill patients, (2) the fact that mentally ill patients are different and easily distinguished from normal people, (3) the causes of the illness including disturbances in the nervous system as well as a lack of will power, and (4) preventive aspects such as for example when a person has a problem, it is better for him or her to concentrate on pleasant activities and not to think too much about the problem.

Regarding authoritarianism, it can be seen in figure 1 that there was a nonsignificant initial difference between the groups under study, the experiential group rating somewhat higher in the scoring. Both experiential and theoretical groups tend to achieve identical results in their global scores by the end of the experience (fig. 2). On the other hand, the theoretical groups move from a greater dispersion in their scoring on authoritarianism to a lesser one, representing a more uniformed scoring among the individuals (fig. 1, 2).

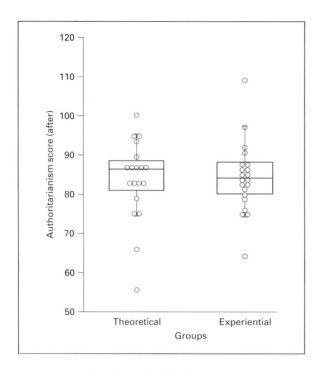

Fig. 2. Authoritarianism (after) according to the two groups.

Discussion

As a result of the group sessions medical students increased their scoring in the authoritarianism dimension. However, that dimension did not change significantly in the experiential groups exposed to dynamic sensitization. The formative groups, which were dedicated to discussing psychiatric cases, experienced a more substantial increase in this rating.

These results agree well with the before-after design studies of medical students following a 6-week formative training program in psychiatry performed by Angoustinus et al. [33], who report an increase in authoritarianism. A more medical conception of mental illness in students was reported too in that study, which does not appear in our present research although it does in previous ones. Yllá et al. [13] report a more substantial increase in authoritarianism in control groups than in experiential groups, in another study carried out with medical students in our department. All these findings are consistent with previous reports of studies carried out among professionals in the field of mental health following a program of group sensitization [9].

As can be seen in figures 1 and 2, the theoretical group which studied psychiatric case histories and whose subjects presented more disperse initial scores became more homogeneous at the end of the experience. As could be expected in this and other formative experiences a greater uniformity of criteria appears. Authoritarianism increases according to other studies among students who were in psychiatric training (formative experiences) [33]. Nevertheless, it is important to point out that the authoritarianism dimension did not change significantly in the experiential group in contrast to the theoretical group. This finding is probably related to the different approach towards mental illness produced in this kind of groups of dynamic sensitization, where personal experience may influence the understanding of the illness.

Our findings could support the idea that with 'classical pedagogical methods' a more uniform and authoritarian attitude is achieved. The group sensitization experiences could preserve this increase of authoritarianism since it makes easy the reflection and knowledge of their psychiatric contents and possible difficulties in the subjects.

The limited number of cases involved in this study suggests that caution should be exercised in regarding these results as conclusive. Consequently this study should be considered as the preliminary phase of a study of a larger scope that would assess the stability or instability of the changes brought about. It should also be remembered that the attitude with its three components, cognitive, affective and behavioral, is difficult to modify in such a short time.

Conclusion

In this article we present findings related to changes of attitude towards mental illness of second-year medical students after group sessions. The students were assigned to two kinds of groups. Experimental groups, where dynamic sensitization techniques of group psychotherapy were applied, and theoretical discussion groups, where psychiatric cases were discussed.

The OMI-R adaptation of Cohen and Struening's questionnaire OMI has been used to measure such attitudes both before and after participation in those groups. Authoritarianism, one of the five dimensions of the OMI-R test, was the dimension which was most substantially altered experiencing an overall increase.

References

1 Lieberman MA, Yalom ID, Miles MB: Encounter Groups: First Facts. New York, Basic Books, 1973.
2 Yalom ID: The Theory and Practice of Group Psychotherapy. New York, Basics Books, 1975.
3 Oppenheimer BT: Short-term small group intervention for college freshmen. J Couns Psychol 1984; 31:45–53.
4 Mackenzie KR: When to recommend group treatment. Int J Group Psychother 1986;36:207–211.
5 Mackenzie KR: Introduction to Time-Limited Group Psychotherapy. Washington, American Psychiatry, 1990.
6 Guimón J, Ozámiz A, Viar I: Actitudes de la población ante el consumo terapeutico de psicofármacos. Actas de la VII Reunión de la Sociedad Española de Psiquiatría Biológica, 1980, pp 165–175.
7 Guimón J, González-Pinto A, Sanz C, González M: Efectos terapéuticos en un programa de sensibilización grupal. Psiquis 1988;1:11–28.
8 González-Pinto A, Gomez O, Castillo E, Bulbena A, Yllá L, Guimón J: Ajuste social en un programa de sensibilización grupal. An Psiqu 1992;8:389–397.
9 González-Pinto A, Castillo E, Gomez O, Yllá L, Guimón J: Cambios de actitud ante la enfermedad mental tras un programa de sensibilización grupal. Psiquis 1993;14:139–151.
10 Azima FJ: The clinical efficacy of group psychotherapy. Int J Group Psychother 1982;32:441–444.
11 Toseland RW, Siporin M: When to recommend group treatment. A review of the clinical and the research literature. Int J Group Psychother 1986;36:171–203.
12 Yllá L, Sanz C, González-Pinto A, Guimón J, Garcia N: Actitudes frente a la enfermedad mental y psicopatología mostrada por estudiantes de Medicina en la Universidad del Pais Vasco. Psiquis 1988;4:57–61.
13 Yllá L, González-Pinto A, Guimón J, Castillo E, Garcia N, González M, Burutaran T: Cambios de actitud ante el paciente mental y variaciones de personalidad medidas a través del SCL–90 en estudiantes de Medicina. Actas Luso Esp Neurol Psiquiatr Cienc 1988;16:356–366.
14 Yllá L, González-Pinto A, Galletero JM, Eguiluz I, Totorika K, Iturriaga I: Cambios en los sintomas psicopatológicos y en la actitud ante la enfermedad mental en estudiantes de Medicina. Actas Soc Esp Psiquiatr Biol 1991;16:430–433.
15 Yllá L, González-Pinto A, Eguiluz I, Zupiria X, Iturriaga I: Aplicación en estudiantes de medicina del cuestionario de Zielke para cambios tras procesos grupales. Actas Luso Esp Neurol Psiquiatr Cienc 1993;4:148–157.
16 Janosik EH: A pragmatic approach to group therapy. J Psychiatr Nurs Ment Health Serv 1972;10: 7–11.
17 Mackenzie KR, Dies RR: Core Battery Clinical Outcome Results. New York, American Group Psychotherapy Association, 1982.
18 García Ruiz M, Vazquez S, Fernandez Lopez JA: Actitudes del médico hacia la Psiquiatría en un Hospital General. Psiquis 1991;1:46–52.
19 Yllá L: Estudio psicosocial y Estadístico de la actitud hacia el enfermo mental de la población general de Vizcaya y de la típica de Bermeo Bilbao; doctoral thesis, UPV, 1979.
20 Yllá L, Ozámiz A, Guimón J: Un análisis psicosocial de las actitudes hacia el enfermo mental. Madrid, Asociación española de Neuropsiquiatria. Colección monográfica. Premios nacionales, 1981.
21 Cohen J, Struening EL: Opinions about mental illness. Hospital differences in attitudes for eight occupational groups. Psychol Rep 1965;14:25–26.
22 Struening EL, Cohen J: Factorial invariance and other psychometric characteristics of the five factors about mental illness opinions. Educ Psychol 1963;23:289–298.
23 Ozámis JA: Actitudes hacia las enfermedades mentales en el País Vasco; doctoral thesis, Madrid, 1980.
24 Whitfield W, Winter RD: Psychiatry and general practice: Results of a Surveying of Avon General practitioners. J R Coll Gen Pract 1980;30:682–686.
25 Ayuso JL: Actitudes hacia la Psiquiatría de los médicos en un Hospital General. Actas Luso Esp Neurol Psiquiatr Cienc 1973;2:347–358.

26 Ayuso JL, Calvé A: La Psiquiatría en el Hospital General. Madrid, Paz Montalvo, 1976.

27 Díez Manrique JF: Actitud médica hacia la Unidad Psiquiátrica de un Hospital General y evaluación crítica. Folia Neuropsiquiátr 1979;14:1–4.

28 Lesser IM, Friedmann CT: Attitudes toward medication change among chronically impaired psychiatric patients. Am J Psychiatry 1981;138:801–803.

29 Payn SB: Group pharmacotherapy for withdrawn schizophrenic patients. Can Psychiatr Assoc J 1978;23:97–98.

30 Eguiluz JI: Evolución actitudinal y clínica de pacientes esquizofrénicos a través de su participación en grupos de medicación; doctoral thesis, Biblioteca de la Facultad de Medicina, Bilbao, Lejona, 1987.

31 O'Mahony PO: An investigation of change in medical student's conceptualization of psychiatric patients due to short training course in psychiatry. Med Educ 1979;13:103–110.

32 Roman PM, Floyd HH: Social acceptance of psychiatric illness and psychiatric treatment. Soc Psychiatry 1981;16:21–29.

33 Angoustinus M, Schader G, Chynoweth R, Reid M: Medical students' attitudes towards psychiatry: A conceptual shift. Psychol Med 1985;15:671–678.

34 Clarke L: The effects of training and social orientation on attitudes towards psychiatric treatments. J Adv Nurs 1989;14:485–493.

35 Zwiebel A: Changing educational counsellors' attitudes toward mental retardation: Comparison of two measurement techniques. Int J Rehabil Res 1987;10:383–389.

36 Balint M: El médico, el paciente y la enfermedad. Buenos Aires, Libros Básicos, 1986.

37 Foulkes SH: Psicoterapia Grupo-Analítica. Método y principios. Barcelona, Gedisa, 1986.

38 Madianos MG, Madianos D, Vlachanikolis J, Stefanis CN: Attitudes towards mental illness in the Athens area: Implications for community mental health intervention. Acta Psychiatr Scand 1987; 75:158–165.

39 Shokoohi J, Retish PN: Attitudes of Chinese and American male students towards mental illness. Int J Soc Psychiatry 1991;37:192–200.

40 Rodriguez Claudio R: Comparación de actitudes de estudiantes de medicina brasileños y españoles hacia la enfermedad mental. Actas Luso Esp Neurol Psiquiatr Cienc 1987;20:30–41.

41 Keane MC: Acceptance versus rejection: Nursing student attitudes about mental illness. Perspect Psychiatry Care Attitudes 1991;27:13–18.

42 Wilkinson L, Hill MA, Welna JP, Birkenbend GK: SYSTAT for windows: Statistics, version 5. Evanston, SYSTAT, 1992.

Prof. Luis Yllá, Departamento de Neurociencias, Seccion Psiquiatría,
Universidad del País Vasco (UPV), E–48940 Lejona, Vizcaya (Spain)
Tel./Fax +34 44 436 488

Guimón J, Fischer W, Sartorius N (eds): The Image of Madness. The Public Facing Mental
Illness and Psychiatric Treatment. Basel, Karger, 1999, pp 138–142

Stigmatization and Destigmatization: The Point of View of Psychiatric Patients and Their Families

Madeleine Pont

GRAAP, Lausanne, Switzerland

The principal aim of the association I run is to change people's image of psychiatric illness. For years I have been working to identify and understand the mechanisms of stigmatization as well as taking action to try to demystify madness so that people can learn to live with it and make something useful out of it, both for themselves and for others. In order to illustrate my thoughts on this theme, I will draw from my own practical experience of the last few years.

It was the difficulty individuals found in bearing the stigmata of their madness that led to the creation of the GRAAP, Groupe d'accueil et d'action psychiatrique – a support and action group for people with psychiatric problems. Ten years ago, I proposed to a group of 9 psychiatric patients and their families, who came for consultations to the social service where I was working, that they should get together to exchange their experiences of madness. More often than not, the discussions turned towards the reputation of their illness. Some even went so far as to say that they felt that the effect of this reputation did them more harm than the illness itself! Following on from this we decided to continue our meetings, to keep a journal of them and to declare to whoever would listen that we did not see ourselves in the way that society saw mad people.

Let us call a spade a spade. Behind terms like mental illness, psychiatric hospital or psychiatry there lies the word 'madness' with all the images that go with it. Whatever we or our families may have experienced – be it suicide, depression, hallucinations, or the impression that we were an incarnation of the Messiah or Hitler, or the fact that we have been diagnosed as being psychotic, anorexic, schizophrenic, hebephrenic or any other of these barbaric terms – from the moment we have been to see a psychiatrist, we are branded as being mad. Some of the members of our group dared not even go out of the house for fear that the words mad or the name of the university psychiatric hospital were actually written all over their face. Let us accept that the words mad and madness have to become an integral part of our everyday life. So let us continue to call a spade a spade, since after all a spade is not a bulldozer!

What Does the Label of Madness Conjure Up?

In the first place, the general public links madness with violence, dangerousness, sadism. You just have to look at the newspapers to see headlines such as, 'Nutcase Throws Furniture out of Window' or 'Maniac on Balcony Shoots Indiscriminately at Passersby' or 'In a Fit of Madness, a Lawyer Goes into Church and Kills the Priest'.

The second image evoked by madness is that of the simpleton – the person who wanders about aimlessly, muttering inaudibly to himself or herself, eyes fixed on the ground. This is your 'loony' or 'village idiot'. There is often confusion between physical and mental handicap here. A further image is that of the eccentric, who is in no way malicious, but is often referred to as 'a real character', 'a bit of a nutcase', 'not all there', 'crazy'.

The public view of psychiatric illness is undifferentiated. It does not understand such illness and is afraid of it. In addition, only the more sensational aspects of it tend to stick in the mind – a fact that is preyed upon and abused by some sectors of the press (cinema and television included). This type of information merely serves to increase the general fear by only showing the extreme, spectacular aspects of madness. This view and these attitudes end up by isolating, excluding and rejecting mental illness as if, in losing his or her reason, a madman or madwoman ceases to be a human being and turns into some sort of animal or even vegetable.

So why do these attitudes exist? Why is there such stigmatization associated with an illness? And why is it so difficult to consider madness to be just like any other illness?

To try and understand this we would need to analyze the subject in depth, taking into account such disciplines as human psychology, history, sociology and so on. Such an analysis is impossible to undertake within the framework of this contribution. Instead, I propose to take a look at the situation as regards stigmatization here and now – today and in our own region. Let me give you some examples.

'No, Madam, it's impossible to rent you these premises. You must understand that times are hard in the real estate business, and we have our reputation to look after. The presence of an association of psychiatric patients would lower the value of the property.' That was the reply I received from an insurance company 2 years ago when I was looking for new premises for the GRAAP. I would just like to add that next door to the premises that interested us, in the same building, a sex shop was in business!

At the same time, a social institution refused to rent us large premises intended for community use for fear that our members would upset the local residents. A number of health insurance companies have just announced that they will no longer offer psychiatric treatment in private wards as an insurance option.

Recently, the Department of Internal Affairs and Public Health in the canton of Vaud began considering a report dealing with the future orientation of public health in the canton. When we asked the departmental head why our association did not feature on the list of consulted organizations he replied without the slightest hesitation that psychiatry had no place in the report, but that he would send us a copy of it for our information. And indeed, this report on the future of public health in our canton contains not a single word on psychiatry! Or rather, there is one mention of it. One finding of a survey carried out throughout Switzerland stated that in the canton of Vaud 25% of the male population and 30% of the female population are reported as having a low level of mental health!

A specialized journal in our area, in publicizing our congress, illustrated its text with an individual holding a funnel upside-down – a sure sign of its contempt for madness.

Parents of adolescents suffering from psychiatric disorders have for some time been asking that the unit which looks after that age group be transferred from the psychiatric hospital to the university hospital, which is the principal general hospital of the region.

Not so long ago – and for all I know it may still be the case – the USA would not grant an entry visa, even a tourist visa, if it is apparent that an individual was suffering from a psychiatric illness.

It is not necessary to give further examples. There is no shortage of work for us to do! Shame, guilt, the silence that surrounds mental illness or a period spent in a psychiatric hospital – all prove that the taboos still exist. Being made fun of, jeered at, treated with scorn, humiliated or rejected are the current types of stigmata that condemn mad people. 'We mad people…' was the way one of our members expressed herself to the local press a few years ago, provoking consternation among the public and a debate within our association.

To stand up in public and state that we have experienced or are experiencing madness, to talk about it without shame or guilt – or without making a big deal out of it either – that is what the GRAAP has been working towards for 10 years, trying to change the image of mental illness. For us this demystification has been no small affair. We have been involved in programs of action on ourselves, with the local community and involving society in general.

In our group meetings we have talked about our experiences, wept about our periods of anxiety, laughed about our moments of delirium, rebelled together against doctors who refused to tell us their diagnosis of our illnesses or who were only willing to listen to their own opinion about our state of health. We swore to teach a lesson to one psychiatrist who insisted that our medication was her business and her business alone and we claimed the right to have our own say in our treatment.

In addition, these illnesses often brought us face to face with death and we were inevitably confronted with the question: what is the point of life after all?

As time went on, our meetings became full of dreams of a society where love, peace, beauty, song, poetry and harmony reigned supreme. We all shared an ideal and were deeply saddened, wounded even, by the reality of our day-to-day existence.

We felt good when we were together, joined by something like benign complicity. Little by little our discussions led us to a better understanding of our illnesses. We could tame them, control them. And when Pascal told us one evening, 'In five years of psychotherapy I haven't spoken so much as I have in one evening here', we became aware that our discussions gave out an energy that was almost tactile.

Whilst we may have realized just how fragile we were, we were no longer ashamed of our illnesses. Through solidarity and friendship we had been able to build up new confidence in ourselves, our plans and our ideals. We felt a strong urge to go on and do things together, involve ourselves in an attempt to put our ideas and points of view to good use in a broader framework.

Today we are a group of over 600 members. We work to establish a society in which values such as solidarity, responsibility and mutual support take precedence over material values. But we are not content to merely sketch out a plan for this society. Based on our principles, we have undertaken a number of different types of action in answer to the basic needs expressed by our members.

And so we – patients and their families together – have set up a number of joint-management projects in relationship with partners from various spheres of the economy, from the political arena and from the areas of public health and social affairs. So far these amount to two reception and support centers, a restaurant, a café, training centers for psychiatric patients, self-help and discussion groups, a publishing unit, a social and legal service and an annual congress which brings together specialists, the general public and of course patients and their families.

For the first 3 years of our existence, all work was done on a voluntary basis. Today in 1997 we have 21 salaried employees, 22 posts for unemployed people who no longer receive unemployment benefit and 50 posts occupied by 200 mentally ill people receiving a disability pension. Our annual budget is nearly two million Swiss francs.

We have just held our annual congress based on the theme, 'Are We All Going Mad?' The congress was attended by about 20 journalists together with 520 members of the general public, patients, families and professionals and they were able to listen to sober and serious presentations about madness, its history, its diagnosis and its treatment. They were able to ask themselves questions on the meaning of madness in our society and on what the role of the state should be. Through numerous personal accounts given by people who live with and deal with madness, those present at the congress could experience at first hand the madness that exists in all of us.

This type of action, where we tackle the question of madness openly amongst ourselves, gives us the courage, strength and confidence to talk about it in public. Paradoxically, when one of our members speaks publicly about his madness and of what he does as an active member of the GRAAP, a definite wave of solidarity, admiration and respect can be felt and the negative image of the illness suffers a rude shock. Madness takes on a more human aspect. Shame and guilt change sides.

A union delegate and several journalists made the following remark to us at the congress: 'We have been most impressed by the recognition you receive from the authorities.' We were pleased to hear this and we are honored to play the role of court jester.

Through these various types of action, we the mad men and women, prove that we are citizens in our own right, responsible, able to lead our own lives and be useful to society as a whole. The GRAAP expects nothing less than this conviction from each of its members.

Mrs. M. Pont, Director, GRAAP, Rue de la Borde 23,
CH–1018 Lausanne (Switzerland)
Tel. +41 21 647 16 00, Fax +41 61 647 16 03

Guimón J, Fischer W, Sartorius N (eds): The Image of Madness. The Public Facing Mental Illness and Psychiatric Treatment. Basel, Karger, 1999, pp 143–151

....

Use and Misuse of Pharmacological Substances: The Question of Noncompliance[1]

J. Guimón, W. Fischer, D. Goerg, E. Zbinden

Department of Psychiatry, University Hospital, Geneva, Switzerland

If the image of psychiatry itself varies considerably according to psychosociological variables, the same is true of the public image of psychiatric treatment, especially in the minds of patients. Bias against certain types of treatment, in particular psychotropic medication, diminishes compliance. It is the source of abundant criticism as well as the cause of a number of lawsuits brought against psychiatrists.

In this chapter, we shall discuss questions dealing with the consumption of and compliance with psychotropic drug treatment and the means at the psychiatrist's disposal to dispel problems arising from noncompliance.

Consumption of Psychotropic Drugs

Extent of Consumption

Studies on psychotropic drug consumption [2] have revealed the frequency of consumption of different types of medication and the determining factors behind this consumption.

At the international level and especially with regard to the frequency of psychotropic drug consumption, studies carried out in Australia [3] and in Sweden [4, 5] must be underlined. These studies indicated that frequency was situated at between 6 and 15% in the general population. This percentage of psychotropic drug users in the general public was borne out by a more recent

---

[1] This chapter has been adapted, with notable modifications, from the text appearing under the heading 'Us et abus des traitements biologiques' in Guimón [1].

study by Takala et al. [6] in Finland: 4.3% of men and 4% of women were using psychotropic medication at the time of the survey. In France, 11.3% of subjects 18 years and older regularly consumed (at least once a week for a minimum of 6 months) at least one psychotropic drug; the rate of regular consumption was higher for women (13.7%) than for men (8.6%) [7].

In Switzerland, two major studies were carried out. The first, undertaken by the Institute of Social and Preventive Medicine at the University of Zurich, also dealt widely with problems linked with prescription drug abuse in the general population [8, 9]. The drug classification used in that study does not permit a direct comparison between its results and those obtained in other studies. However it would appear that the intake of psychotropic drugs by the public was, as in other countries, low: during the 15-day period prior to the survey, 6–7% of subjects had taken medically prescribed sedatives or tranquilizers and 1.1% stimulants.

In the second study, carried out by the Swiss Institute for the Prevention of Alcoholism, it was found that 2% of the general population took sedatives or tranquilizers daily and 3.6% stimulants [10]. As in other studies, it was noted that women used psychotropic drugs more than men: 2.4% had a daily intake of sedatives or tranquilizers and 4.3% stimulants as against 1.6 and 2.8% of men. An increase in consumption with increasing age was also observed. Neither of these studies dealt with data on neuroleptics and antidepressants. The results of a recent 'Swiss Health Survey' confirmed these results; 11.8% of women and 5.7% of men had taken psychiatric medication (major and minor tranquilizers, sleeping pills) in the week prior to the survey and this consumption was linked to age [11].

Determining Factors in the Consumption of Psychotropic Medication

Several studies measured not only the consumption of psychotropic drugs, but its relationship to the physical and mental state of health of the interviewees. Other parameters (medical consumption in general, emotional lability, life events, social problems, alcohol, tobacco, coffee consumption, sociodemographic, family and professional characteristics) were also considered. These studies showed that beyond the already mentioned incidence of gender and age, strong correlations existed between certain health circumstances and psychiatric morbidity.

It thus appeared that subjects placed in very particular health circumstances considerably increased their recourse to psychotropic medication. This was the case for Alzheimer family member caregivers, 30% of whom took psychotropic medication [12]. This percentage of consumption was also very high when subjects who presented psychiatric symptoms evoked by a questionnaire on mental health were taken into consideration [13]: 20.1% of men and

19.3% of women suffering from mental disorders took psychotropic medication. It should be pointed out that these subjects generally had markedly higher rates of consumption in all categories of medication.

Guimón et al. [14] confirmed these results in their study of patients (n = 900) of general practitioners in the Basque Country. Only 2% of these patients presented a psychiatric diagnosis made by their general practitioner. However, 42.8% showed signs of a psychiatric symptomatology exceeding the limit set by Goldberg [13]. With regard to medicine consumption, 31% of patients took medication which acted on the central nervous system of which 59.9% was self-prescribed; 22.9% took medication despite a lack of any mental pathology as evaluated on Goldberg's scale. This consumption, therefore, supported the theory of self-medication as a remedy against psychological distress which had been neither diagnosed nor treated in an adequate manner.

However, the differences in psychotropic drug consumption were far greater when the subjects' own personal experience with psychiatry and psychiatric treatment was taken into account. Thus Weyerer and Dilling [15] found the following percentages in psychotropic drug consumers classified by the type of psychiatric treatment: no treatment 5.4%, hospital treatment only 20.0%, outpatient only 31.3% and hospital treatment + outpatient 63.0%. In consequence, in addition to mental disturbance itself, other factors such as the subjects' history of successive treatments seemed to be linked to a high consumption of psychotropic medication.

Correlations which were weaker, but still significant, were also observed with somatic morbidity. But there again, the everyday effects of illness seemed a consequential factor in the overconsumption of psychotropic medication. Principally concerned were chronic health problems: headaches, epilepsy, hypertension [16], disability and invalidity [17] and the subject's own negative feelings about his or her state of health at the time of the survey [12, 15]. The covariation between psychotropic drug overconsumption and frequent recourse to the health care system (an important incidence of medical consultations) would seem to be contingent on the serious health problems we have just mentioned [12, 15]. Furthermore, the overconsumption of psychotropic drugs appeared to be linked to the abuse of alcohol [17] and tobacco [16].

In addition to age and gender, other social factors influenced, in a significant manner, the overconsumption of psychotropic drugs. A lower educational level and a lower socioprofessional level were some of these factors [4, 7, 12, 18]. The 'Swiss Health Survey' showed that education and income influenced consumption of medication in general and, in particular, that of psychiatric drugs [11]. To a lower level of education corresponded a higher consumption of medication. A lower income acted in the same way. A profile of the typical consumer of psychiatric medication was thus (even more so than for the archetype of the consumer of medication in general), an elderly woman with a low level of income and a low level of education.

Finally, subjects who were disenfranchised or had left the workplace (early retirement, incapacity to work, housewives) also consumed more psychotropic drugs [17, 19].

Zbinden and Gognalons-Nicolet [11] have looked into the very selective social circumstances involved in the use of this type of medication.

Compliance Question

The question of attitudes of the general public toward psychiatric treatment and particularly towards psychotropic medication was recently dealt with at a symposium that we organized within the context of the European Congress of the World Psychiatric Association which was held in Geneva in 1997; this question was reviewed in depth and the subject is developed in this book. The specific question of public attitudes toward psychotropic drugs is the object of an article contained herein; the different aspects dealt with have close ties to compliance [20].

Factors Determining Poor Compliance

Various studies carried out in controlled clinical settings, which we have recently discussed [2], pointed to patients' low level of compliance with psychotropic drugs. According to a review of the literature done by Jamison [21] concerning tricyclic antidepressant drugs, noncompliance rated at between 32 and 76%. However, it decreased appreciably when medicinal treatment was accompanied by psychotherapy and then the incidence of noncompliance was between 10 and 33%. The seven studies published concerning treatment with lithium showed a rate of noncompliance that varied between 18 and 47%. As for treatment with neuroleptics, oral administration in outpatient settings resulted in a 10–76% rate of noncompliance [22]. Comparable results came out of a study on crisis intervention and the long-term evolution of depressive patients [23]. In particular, patients who were characterized by a better therapeutic alliance and a better grasp of their disorder at the end of the crisis intervention also proved to be more compliant in the long term. This higher compliance implied a better evolution during the 2 years which followed. As was already shown by Frank et al. [24], the results of these different studies showed the fundamental role information and education play in increasing patient compliance with treatment and, thus, favoring in particular their compliance with psychotropic drugs.

Negative attitudes towards psychotropic medication had a correlation with poor compliance, as was shown in the study we carried out in Geneva [20].

In a study on patients suffering serious psychiatric disorders, Draine and Solomon [25] showed that the following factors were significantly associated with more positive attitudes towards drugs: increased age, a less serious symptomatology and a larger scope of daily activities which implied social interaction. Taking part in social activities – one of the practical goals of rehabilitation – also constituted an important aid to compliance with psychiatric treatment in general and with medicinal treatment in particular [26, 27].

Other studies have looked more specifically at the prescription practices of therapists, particularly general practitioners: posology, mode of administration, optimal dosage so as to decrease as much as possible the secondary effects which are largely responsible for noncompliance and which occur principally at the beginning of pharmacological treatment.

DiMatteo et al. [28] considered noncompliance not as an irrational act, but rather as a rational choice based on the following two main factors. It was determined, firstly, by the patient's lack of faith in the usefulness and effectiveness of the drug and by the fact that its benefits might be judged to be insufficient when compared to the disadvantages caused by its cost and the inconvenience associated with compliance. Secondly, it resulted from difficulty in complying with the prescription itself as well as because of a lack of family and social support for the patient. In consequence, an important task of the therapist is to better inform patients and negotiate the prescription of pharmacological treatment with them.

Similar conclusions could be made in the study by Lorenc and Branthwaite [29], according to which seven parameters were significantly and independently linked to strong compliance: adequate knowledge of how treatment was set up, belief in the importance of closely following medical prescriptions, low resentment of time spent waiting to see the doctor, absence of fear of illness, ability to read the label on the bottle, understanding what the physician has said and the fact that the patient does not live alone.

Angermeyer and Matschinger [30] found that the patient's incentive to comply with a prescription was greater when he/she believed the therapy to be effective. In contrast, when a patient doubted the beneficial effects of treatment, they also doubted psychiatric knowledge with regard to etiology, to prognosis as well as to adequate therapy for the disorder. Thus, a low level of compliance in patients and their entourage constituted a quasi-unavoidable consequence.

In a slightly different perspective, Goerg et al. [31], addressed the question of dropping out of psychiatric treatment through a unilateral decision of the patient that can be considered as global noncompliance. This study was carried out at the Department of Psychiatry of the University of Geneva among new patients and their therapists. It showed that treatment dropout probability was higher when patients did not share the same values as the psychiatric institution and when little congruence existed between the attitudes of patients and those of therapists, both with regard to defining problems and to treatment expectations. The fact that a certain number of patients kept up treatment despite an absence of congruence must be analyzed in structural terms (conformity, submissiveness, various pressures) rather than in cultural ones (values, normative expectations).

Techniques to Improve Compliance

It is obviously necessary to spearhead an effort aimed at modifying bias in the general public in relation to the therapeutic use of psychopharmacological substances. Media campaigns on the effects of these products, their indications and counterindications could help to decrease prejudice which is prevalent, as we have seen, among persons of a low cultural level.

We should undoubtedly begin by modifying the attitudes of care-providers themselves. Bury et al. [32] showed that a significant change occurred in attitudes toward psychopharmacological substances among medical students before and after their courses in psychiatry. But they did not ascertain whether this modification endured in their subsequent careers. A recent study among medical students [33] showed that stereotypes, which were comparable at the beginning of medical studies to those held by the general public, decreased progressively with advancing knowledge.

Although we believe it possible to modify certain cognitive aspects of attitudes toward these products, we are more pessimistic with regard to the possibility of influencing all the other aspects which are based on affective reactions and which are often unconscious and very difficult to modify. On this topic, it is important for the reader to remember the celebrated study which related the failure of an attempt to modify the attitudes on mental illness of citizens of a town in North America [34]. The campaign, waged through various media over a period of several months, did not succeed in modifying public attitudes in an appreciable manner. To the contrary, it elicited some irritation in those persons it sought to influence.

Effectively, a rejection of medication may result from deep psychological factors arising in the relationship between the patient and his or her psychiatrist. One example of this consists in the negative placebo effect, which may take the form of collateral symptoms that cannot be explained from a pharmacological point of view [35]. These effects were frequently caused by the patient's deep-seated resistance. Van Putten et al. [36] have shown, for example, that an ego-syntonic sense of psychotic 'grandeur' was the most important factor which distinguished schizophrenic patients showing poor compliance from those with a strong compliance.

In the same way, an excessive tendency to deny illness leads many patients to put up a determined resistance to pharmacotherapy. Other patients are not compliant because of the existence of 'secondary benefits', which cause them to prefer illness to health. These patients might even 'hang on to symptoms' once they have been treated, thereby rendering medication ineffective. Some others refuse medication in order to deny that their illness really exists from a psychiatric point of view.

The prescription of medication by a psychiatrist could, on the other hand, activate an unconscious parental transference which can drive the patient to poor compliance. This is particularly true for patients who have been termed manipulative help rejectors. When psychiatrists adopt an authoritarian tone with these patients, it only contributes to increasing the patient's opposition. Some might even threaten to drop patients who do not comply or they might instill feelings of guilt so that patients only obey in order to avoid offending their psychiatrist. Some psychiatrists might also accept that patients interrupt medication in order to demonstrate how ill they would feel without it [37]. In contrast, some psychotherapists might not prescribe a very necessary medication because they narcissistically fear that it might bring into question the effectiveness of their technique.

Public information is therefore insufficient to improve compliance with medication. This is true to such a degree that a certain number of types of specific intervention have been created. Ciancetta [38] compared the results of a psychotherapeutic program in which the patient was seen individually by a psychiatrist during a half hour every month with a group format in which 7 patients were seen for 75 minutes once a month. The group program was significantly more effective. Pakes [39] obtained, in his study, good results from a nondirective program.

In the same way, one of us examined with Eguiluz et al. [40], within the framework of a controlled study, the evolution of schizophrenic patients who took part in a group program concerned with neuroleptic medication in a day hospital. These patients attended eight semistructured weekly group meetings; their families were also included in a similar program. Their attitudes towards psychotropic medication, their compliance and their clinical evolution were measured at quarterly intervals over a year and compared to those of the control group which did not benefit from any intervention. Medication compliance and BPRS ratings improved significantly more in the experimental group than in the control group. Attitudes towards medication improved similarly in both groups after the 12-month observation period, although during the first 2 months, significantly more in the experimental group. Attitudinal changes were also noticed in the families of patients, both in the experimental group and in the control group.

During a later study with González Torres and Eguiluz [41], we were able to show, through similar techniques, that patients taking part in psychoeducational group therapy presented fewer cases of readmission than those of the control group.

In conclusion, we think that the attempts made to modify attitudes towards psychopharmacological substances require, in addition to the setting up of public education programs, information campaigns aimed at physicians who prescribe these products in order to help them determine a patient's prejudices and how they can be modified.

References

1   Guimón J: La profession de psychiatre. Evolution et devenir. Paris, Masson, 1998.
2   Guimón J, Fischer W, Goerg D, Zbinden E: Médicaments psychotropes et population générale: consommation, attitudes et représentations. Cah Psychiatr 1996;21:229–250.
3   Lockwood A, Berbatis CG: Psychotropic drugs in Australia: Consumption patterns. Med J Aust 1990;153:604–611.
4   Isacson D, Haglund B: Psychotropic drug use in a Swedish community. The importance of demographic and socioeconomic factors. Soc Sci Med 1988;4:477–483.
5   Isacson D, Carsjö K, Haglund B, Smedby B: Psychotropic drug use in a Swedish community. Patterns of individual use during 2 years. Soc Sci Med 1988;3:263–267.
6   Takala J, Ryynanen OP, Lehtovirta E, Turakka H: The relationship between mental health and drug use. Acta Psychiatr Scand 1993;88:256–258.
7   Lempérière T: Epidémiologie de l'usage des psychotropes. Rev Int Psychopathol 1996;21:67–77.
8   Hornung R: Medikamentenabusus in der Schweiz. Suchtprobl Sozialarb 1988;3:111–119.
9   Hornung R: Utilisation et abus de médicaments; in Weiss W (ed): La santé en Suisse. Lausanne, Payot, 1993, pp 261–269.
10 Fahrenkrug H, Müller R: Alkohol und Gesundheit in der Schweiz. Arbeitsberichte der Forschungsabteilung, Schweizerische Fachstelle für Alkoholprobleme, Lausanne, 1989.
11 Zbinden E, Gognalons-Nicolet M: Usage social des médicaments à visée psychologique. Cah Psychiatr 1996;21:219–228.
12 Clipp EC, George LK: Psychotropic drug use among caregivers of patients with dementia. J Am Geriatr Soc 1990;3:227–235.
13 Goldberg DP: The Detection of Psychiatric Illness by Questionnaire. London, Oxford University Press, 1972.
14 Guimón J, Ozamiz A, Ylla L, Echevarria A, Sanjuán C: Automedicacion en poblacion general y en pacientes médicos; in Casas M (ed): Trastornos psiquicos en las toxicomanias. Barcelona, Ediciones en Neurociencias, 1992, pp 341–354.
15 Weyerer S, Dilling H: Psychiatric and physical illness, sociodemographic characteristics, and the use of psychotropic drugs in the community: Results from the Upper Bavarian Field Study. J Clin Epidemiol 1991;3:303–311.
16 Pariente P, Lépine JP, Lellouch J: Self-reported psychotropic drug use and associated factors in a French community sample. Psychol Med 1992;22:181–190.
17 Turrina C, Zimmermann-Tansella C, Micciolo R, Siciliani O: A community survey of psychotropic drug consumption in South Verona: Prevalence and associated variables. Soc Psychiatry Psychiatr Epidemiol 1993;28:40–44.
18 Vazquez-Barquero JL, Diez Manrique JF, Pena C, Arenal Gonzalez A, Cuesta MJ, Artal JA: Patterns of psychotropic drug use in a Spanish rural community. Br J Psychiatry 1989;155:633–641.
19 Fichter MM, Witzke W, Leibl K, Hippius H: Psychotropic drug use in a representative community sample: The Upper Bavarian Study. Acta Psychiatr Scand 1989;80:68–77.

20   Fischer W, Goerg D, Zbinden E, Guimón J: Determining factors and the effects of attitudes towards psychotropic medication; in Guimón J, Fischer W, Sartorius N (eds): The Image of Madness. Basel, Karger, 1999.

21   Jamison KR: Psychological Management of Bipolar Disorders. Pharmacologic Prevention of Recurrence. Consensus Development Conference of Mood Disorders, Washington, 1984.

22   Young JL, Zonana HV, Shepler L: Medication noncompliance in schizophrenia: Codification and update. Bull Am Acad Psychiatry Law 1986;14:105–122.

23   Andreoli A, Frances A, Gex-Fabry M, Aapro N, Gerin P, Dazord A: Crisis intervention in depressed patients with and without DSM-III-R personality disorders. J Nerv Ment Dis 1993;12:732–737.

24   Frank E, Prien RF, Kupfer DJ, Alberts L: Implications of noncompliance on research in affective disorders. Psychopharmacol Bull 1985;1:37–42.

25   Draine J, Solomon P: Explaining attitudes toward medication compliance among a seriously mentally ill population. J Nerv Ment Dis 1994;1:50–54.

26   Bachrach LL: Psychosocial rehabilitation and psychiatry in the care of long-term patients. Am J Psychiatry 1992;149:1455–1463.

27   Cook JA, Hoffschmidt SJ: A comprehensive model of psychosocial rehabilitation; in Flexer RW, Solomon PL (eds): Psychiatric Rehabilitation in Practice. Boston, Andover Medical, 1993, pp 81–97.

28   DiMatteo MR, Reiter RC, Gambone JC: Enhancing medication adherence through communication and informed collaborative choice. Health Commun 1994;4:253–265.

29   Lorenc L, Branthwaite A: Are older adults less compliant with prescribed medication than younger adults? Br J Clin Psychol 1993;32:485–492.

30   Angermeyer MC, Matschinger H: Lay beliefs about schizophrenic disorder: The results of a population survey in Germany. Acta Psychiatr Scand 1994;89(suppl 382):39–45.

31   Goerg D, Zbinden E, Duvanel B: Congruence patients-thérapeutes et dropout en psychiatrie ambulatoire publique. Sci Soc Santé 1990;3:49–71.

32   Bury JA, Villeneuve A, Pires A, Lachance R: Evaluation of the attitude and acquisition of knowledge in psychiatry and psychopharmacology during the non-resident term of study. Vie Méd Can Fr 1973;9:849–854.

33   Hillert A: Attitudes towards psychotropic medication among medical students; in Guimón J, Fischer W, Sartorius N (eds): The Image of Madness. Basel, Karger, 1999.

34   Cumming E, Cumming J: Closed Ranks: An Experiment in Mental Health. Cambridge, Harvard University Press, 1957.

35   Gutheil TG: The psychology of psychopharmacology. Bull Menninger Clin 1982;46:321–330.

36   Van Putten T, Crumpton E, Yale C: Drug refusal in schizophrenia and the wish to be crazy. Arch Gen Psychiatry 1976;33:1443–1446.

37   Book HE: Some psychodynamics of non-compliance. Can J Psychiatry 1987;32:115–117.

38   Ciancetta MD: Individual vs group medication review programs for chronic psychiatry patients; International Dissertation abstracts, part B 44:2, p 603, August 1983.

39   Pakes GE: Group medication counselling conducted by a pharmacist for severely disturbed clients. Hosp Community Psychiatry 1979;4:237–238.

40   Guimón J, Eguiluz I, Bulbena A: Group pharmacotherapy in schizophrenics: Attitudinal and clinical changes. Eur J Psychiatry 1993;3:147–154.

41   Eguiluz I, González Torres MA, Guimón J: Psychoeducational groups in schizophrenic patients; in Guimón J, Fischer W, Sartorius N (eds): The Image of Madness. Basel, Karger, 1999.

José Guimón, Département de Psychiatrie, Hôpitaux Universitaires de Genève,
2, chemin du Petit-Bel-Air, CH–1225 Chêne-Bourg (Switzerland)
Tel. +41 22 305 57 77, Fax +41 22 305 57 99

Guimón J, Fischer W, Sartorius N (eds): The Image of Madness. The Public Facing Mental Illness and Psychiatric Treatment. Basel, Karger, 1999, pp 152–161

....

The Public's Attitude towards Drug Treatment of Schizophrenia

Matthias C. Angermeyer, Herbert Matschinger

Department of Psychiatry, University of Leipzig, Germany

It is generally agreed that noncompliance presents a serious problem in the drug treatment of mental disorder. A number of studies have been carried out in order to identify predictors of noncompliant behavior. Up to the present, attention has been concentrated mainly on the characteristics of the patient (e.g. his social status, personality, degree of insight), the type and severity of the mental disturbance, and, finally, the wanted and unwanted effects of drug therapy [1]. The social context of psychiatric treatment, on the other hand, has hardly ever been the subject of research. The influence which opinions of the lay public with regard to the 'right' treatment and popular beliefs about the benefits and risks of drug treatment in general might have on the patients' compliance has largely been ignored.

We therefore set out to investigate by means of a representative survey the attitude of the German public towards psychotropic drug treatment. We wanted to explore what people's treatment preferences are. To what extent is psychotropic medication recommended or advised against as compared with other treatment modalities? We also intended to learn more about the arguments being used to substantiate the support for or rejection of drug treatment. Finally, our goal was to identify possible determinants of treatment choice, focusing on two factors which, in our view, may be of importance in determining whether a particular treatment is recommended or not: people's appraisal of the disorder in question and the assessment of the effectiveness of the treatment.

In this paper we will concentrate on the attitude towards drug treatment of schizophrenia as, with this disorder, the problem of noncompliance is considered to be particularly severe. According to a synopsis published by Young et al. [2], noncompliance with oral neuroleptic medication is to be observed in 10–76% of patients in outpatient treatment.

Method

During 1990 we carried out a representative survey in the Federal Republic of Germany, in cooperation with the Centre for Surveys, Methods and Analyses (ZUMA) in Mannheim and the Association for Marketing, Communications and Social Research (GFM-GETAS) in Hamburg. Our sample included all German nationals who, at the time of the survey, were at least 18 years old and living in private households. In the western part of Germany we conducted a total of 2,118 interviews, and in the eastern part we conducted 980 interviews. The response rates were 71.9 and 67.4%, respectively.

The fully structured interview began with the presentation of a vignette depicting a case of schizophrenic psychosis, major depression or panic disorder with agoraphobia. These three disorders were chosen because each represented at the time the typical indication for one of the three main groups of psychotropic drugs: neuroleptics, antidepressants and minor tranquillizers. The symptoms described in the vignettes fulfilled the DSM-III-R criteria for the respective disorders. Our total sample was divided into subsamples of equal size which were each presented with only one vignette.

Following presentation of the vignette, one of the questions that we asked our respondents was which method of treatment they would either recommend or advise against for the particular pathological behavior described. Using a 5-point scale ranging from 'would highly recommend' to 'would not recommend at all', respondents were asked to provide their assessment of the different treatment methods offered by us which, in addition to psychopharmacotherapy, also included psychotherapy and one 'alternative' method, natural remedies. If those questioned had chosen psychotropic medication, or, on the other hand, had advised against this form of treatment, they were then also explicitly asked why they had endorsed this form of treatment. All explanations by respondents concerning their choice of treatment were recorded by the interviewer and later underwent a content analysis.

In order to examine the influence of a person's overall value orientation on his/her assessment of specific treatment modalities, respondents in the western part of Germany were given a list of 18 behaviors developed by Maag [3]. On the basis of an 8-point scale they were then asked to indicate their opinion about the social desirability of these behaviors. The 18 items were then subjected to a maximum-likelihood factor analysis with oblique rotation yielding the following three dimensions, which largely correspond to those published by Maag [3]. (1) Liberal values (eigenvalue 5.8; explained variance 32.0%): treating all people equally (factor loading 0.76), being just (0.70), dealing fairly with others (0.69), showing tolerance (0.65), removing social differences between individuals (0.62), solving problems by compromise (0.53), increasing participation in decision-making processes (0.43). (2) Traditional values (eigenvalue 1.5; explained variance 8.4%): accomplishing one's tasks (factor loading 0.71), being conscientious (0.71), trying one's best (0.68), being punctual (0.68), valuing wealth (0.63), being careful (0.62). (3) Modern values (eigenvalue 1.2; explained variance 6.8%): enjoying life (factor loading 0.64), doing as you please (0.56), seeking self-realization (0.54), being independent (0.54).

The ideas of those questioned about the causes of the disorder described in the vignettes were recorded using a catalogue of 30 potential etiological factors and a 5-point-scale which ranged from 'definitely a cause' to 'definitely not a cause'. They were asked to record the weighting they assigned to each of the possible causes. Out of this pool of items we chose two to represent each of the following areas: biological (brain disease, hereditary factors), psychological (distinguishing between psychodynamic influences, unconscious conflict, stressful life events) and personality deficiencies (lack of will power, drug abuse), societal (exploitation in industrial society, deterioration of living conditions) and supernatural (horoscope, possession by evil spirits). Our choice was based on a principal variable analysis [4].

The prognosis of the disorder assumed by our respondents was assessed using an ordinal scale with five categories representing the main types of course actually taken by mental illness as follows: total healing, complete remission with possibility of relapse, partial remission, chronic persistence of symptoms and chronic state with steady deterioration.

The general attitude to drug therapy was examined using eight items. In particular we asked whether 'chemical' agents or 'natural' medicines were preferred, how high the threshold to their taking medicine was and how dangerous they considered drug treatment to be. Those questioned expressed their views on each using a 5-point scale ranging from 'totally agree' to 'totally disagree'. These eight items were subjected to a nonlinear principal component analysis with rank one restriction [5, 6]. In the following analysis, the object scores of the first principal axis will be used.

Eleven items were used to record the appraisal of the effects of psychotropic drugs. Five statements proposed beneficial aspects (efficacy, reliability, rapid response, method of choice for severe mental disturbances, and advantages outweighing disadvantages). Three items dealt with criticism of drug treatment (not a treatment of the cause, effects only sedative, no solution to problems). Three further items described unwanted effects (development of dependency, production of cerebral damage and worsening of the condition of the patient). Again, a nonlinear principal component analysis was carried out and the first principal axis will be used in our analysis.

Results

Treatment Recommendations

Figure 1 shows the percentage of respondents who endorsed or rejected the two most important established psychiatric treatment methods, i.e. pharmacotherapy and psychotherapy, for schizophrenic disorder. It also shows the number of respondents who had either recommended or advised against natural remedies, the 'alternative' method. What stands out is a very marked unwillingness to recommend drug therapy which was in fact recommended by only a fifth and rejected by twice as many of those questioned. Psychotherapy was seen completely differently. Over half of those questioned recommended it. Only every tenth respondent rejected it. The alternative method was recommended by a quarter, this being a larger proportion than that recommending drug treatment. The pattern found is similar for both parts of Germany.

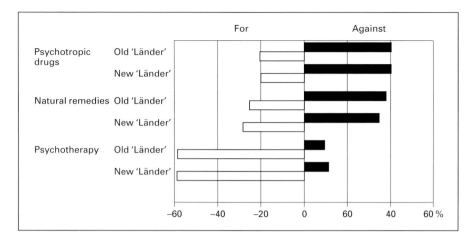

Fig. 1. Recommendations by the lay public concerning the treatment of schizophrenic disorders.

Subjective Reasons for Recommending or Advising against Drug Treatment

The most important argument against the use of psychotropic drugs, cited by almost 40% of the respondents, was the undesirable side effects of the medication. In particular, the risk of addiction motivated a large number of respondents (1 in 6) to warn against the use of psychotropic drugs. One fourth of the respondents criticized the use of psychotropic drugs on the basis that psychopharmacotherapy represents only a treatment of symptoms rather than working on a causal level. As those questioned felt that drug treatment is simply aimed at calming the patient and thus would only help to repress underlying problems, this therapeutic approach seemed little desirable.

Less frequently, respondents also criticized the assumed ineffectiveness of the drugs, or their argument was based on a general dislike of medicines. In some cases they also argued that such treatment was not indicated as the person described in the vignette was either not ill at all, or at least not seriously ill (fig. 2).

Among the small group consisting of those subjects who supported the use of psychopharmacotherapy, the most frequently cited reason given was the sedative effect of these drugs, with one fourth of respondents basing their treatment recommendations on this aspect. One in 6 subjects interviewed qualified their arguments in favor of psychotropic drugs by pointing out that they should be used in combination with psychotherapy. Only 15% recommended drug treatment because of its therapeutic efficacy. Other beneficial effects of psychotropic medication, e.g. its palliative and supportive effect,

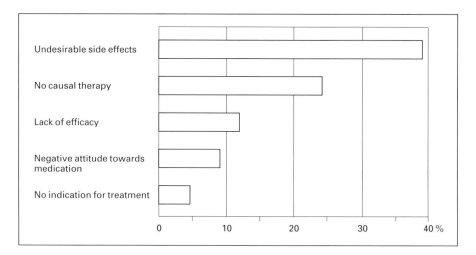

Fig. 2. The five most frequently cited arguments against drug treatment of schizophrenic disorders (n = 374).

were mentioned just as frequently in support of this form of treatment. Approximately 10% of participants recommended this type of treatment based on their overall positive attitude towards psychotropic medication (fig. 3).

Determinants of Treatment Recommendations

After having presented the arguments cited by our respondents in favor of or against drug treatment of schizophrenia we will investigate potential determinants of their treatment recommendations. It was our assumption that two factors are of main importance for treatment recommendation: people's appraisal of the disorder in question and the assessment of the effectiveness of the treatment. The choice of treatment ought to depend on the beliefs of the public about the causes of the disorder. Our hypothesis 1 was that people who consider biological factors to be causative should expect better results from drug therapy and so be more likely to recommend it. On the other hand, people who prefer a psychological explanation should expect psychotherapy to be more effective.

As an indicator for people's beliefs about the severity of the disorder, the prognosis with regard to the natural course of the illness was used. Our hypothesis 2 was that people who expect an unfavorable course should tend to recommend a more 'drastic' form of therapy such as drug treatment. Firstly, because this promises to be more effective, and, secondly, because in such cases they might be more prepared to accept the risks associated with it. On

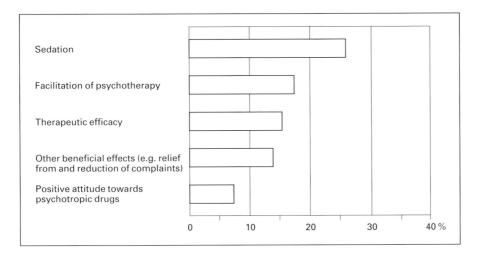

Fig. 3. The five most frequently cited arguments in favor of drug treatment of schizophrenic disorders (n = 189).

the other hand, people who expect a more favorable course should be more inclined to recommend psychotherapy, this seeming to be adequate and associated with a relatively small risk.

As far as assessment by the public of the effects of the different methods is concerned, we have to differentiate between their wanted and unwanted effects. Our hypothesis 3 was that the more the wanted outweigh the unwanted effects, that is the greater the expected benefit and the smaller the costs are thought to be, drug treatment should be recommended with increasing frequency.

As an additional assumption we suggested that the appraisal of the effects of drug treatment should be strongly influenced by the attitude towards drug treatment in general. Our hypothesis 4 was that when those questioned had a favorable attitude towards drug treatment in general, they should tend to assign desirable rather than undesirable effects to psychotropic medication.

All the factors assumed to play a part in the decision for or against drug treatment for mental disorder are also influenced, as we suggested, by people's value orientations. Hence our hypothesis 5 was that people who adhere to 'traditional' views should be more prepared to recommend drug treatment for mental disorder and those with 'liberal' views should tend to reject it.

The hypothesised relationships are shown in figure 4. The model contains three hierarchically ordered sets of variables. The most exogenous variables (first set) are the three factors of a person's overall value orientation; the

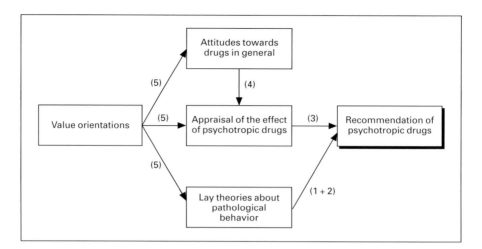

Fig. 4. Determinants of the recommendation of psychotropic medication (the numbers refer to the hypotheses formulated for each path).

second set contains the 10 potential causes, the assumed prognosis of the disorder, the general attitude towards drug therapy as well as the appraisal of the effect of psychotropic drugs. The two variables measuring treatment recommendations are the most endogenous ones. Since we have no theoretical assumptions about the direction of particular effects between the variables of the second set, path coefficients between these variables were restricted to zero. However we know that these variables are correlated, and these correlations somehow have to be considered in the regression equations. In order to obtain a fully saturated explanatory model (no constraints on the effects) despite these restrictions, the covariances of the residual terms of the respective variables are not restricted to zero, but rather are estimated, in this way representing the empirical covariance between the variables of the second set. Thus we did not employ a model in a strict statistical sense.

The results of the path analysis are shown in figure 5. The more those questioned were 'liberally' oriented, the less favorable were their attitudes towards drug treatment in general and the less positive was their appraisal of the effect of psychotropic drugs in particular. By contrast, the more 'traditional' their values were, the more positively they evaluated the effect of psychotropic medication.

There were hardly any relationships between value orientation and lay theory about schizophrenic disorder except for a more marked tendency to deny supernatural influences and to give a more favorable prognosis among those with a stronger attachment to liberal values. Those holding traditional

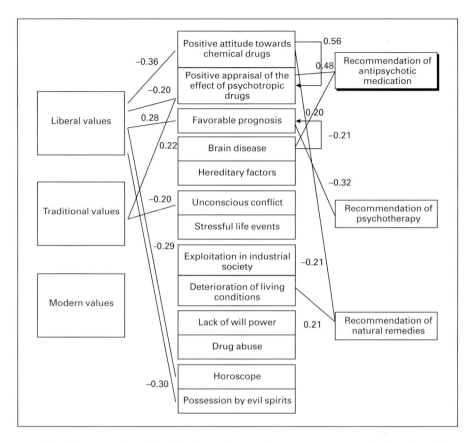

Fig. 5. Structural model of the determinants of treatment recommendations for schizo-phrenia.

values were less prepared to accept that schizophrenic disorders may be caused by unconscious conflicts. The attachment to 'modern values' had no influence at all on the appraisal of drug treatment or on lay theories about causation and prognosis.

The attitude towards drug therapy in general had a marked influence on the assessment of the effectiveness of psychotropic medication. If someone had a favorable opinion as to the effects of these, he/she tended to recommend them for the treatment of schizophrenic disorders. Those who thought that schizophrenia may be due to a brain disease were more willing to recommend drug treatment. All other potential causal factors as well as the assumed progress of the disorder had no influence on the recommendation of this form of treatment.

As one might expect those who are rather in favor of 'chemical' drugs were less inclined to recommend natural remedies. The opposite applies to those who were more ecologically minded ('deterioration of living conditions'). That those respondents who expected the disorder to take a favorable course did hesitate to recommend psychotherapy may at first glance appear rather counterintuitive. As suggested by other findings this may be due to the fact that these people thought that, instead of seeking help from professionals, the person described in the vignette should rather rely on his/her self help potential or his/her support resources.

Discussion

In the general public, psychotropic drug treatment of schizophrenia is met with far more disapproval than approval. It was rejected twice as often as it was recommended. On the other hand, psychotherapy enjoyed a much better reputation. Even the 'alternative' form of treatment tended to be more likely to be recommended than psychotropic drugs. Thus, there is a sharp contrast between the lay public's belief as regards the 'right' treatment of schizophrenia and the opinion of psychiatric experts. In the eyes of the latter, psychotropic medication is the first treatment option in addition to which special forms of psychotherapy are to be applied. Alternative therapies are considered at best useless if not harmful. Remarkably, among the undesirable effects attributed to psychotropic drugs, addiction ranked first, although this is not a risk with neuroleptics. Apparently, people are not able to differentiate between the different classes of psychotropic drugs and lump neuroleptics and benzodiazepines together. This interpretation is also supported by the finding that sedation was the reason most often given for the recommendation of drug treatment of schizophrenia [7].

Of our hypotheses about determinants of treatment choice, only the third and fourth were confirmed by our findings. These are those stating that the more favorable the effects of psychotropic drugs were judged to be, the greater was the preparedness to recommend this form of treatment. As we suggested in our fourth hypothesis, opinions about the effectiveness of psychotropic agents were strongly influenced by the attitude towards drug treatment in general. The other hypotheses were not confirmed. Neither the beliefs about the causation nor the assessment of the prognosis had any influence on the decision to recommend or to advise against drug treatment. Attitudes towards mental illness and opinions about its treatment were influenced by the general attitude, but only to a small extent.

Thus, the model which we formulated at the beginning could only be partially confirmed by our findings. It must also be said that its explanatory power was fairly limited. The standardized residues were all high and less than 10% of the overall variance was explained with the exception of the variable 'assessment of the effectiveness of treatment' where 35% of the variance was accounted for.

References

1 Angermeyer MC: Compliance schizophrener Kranker mit Neuroleptika-Medikation; in Möller HJ (ed): Langzeiterfahrungen mit Glianimon. Cologne, Tropon-Werke, 1991.
2 Young JC, Zonana HV, Shepler L: Medication non-compliance in schizophrenia: Codification and update. Bull Am Acad Psychiatry Law 1986;14:105–122.
3 Maag G: Zur Erfassung von Werten in der Umfrageforschung. Z Soziol 1989;18:313–323.
4 McCabe GP: Principle variables. Technometrics 1984;26:137–144.
5 Gifi A: PRINCALS Users Manual. Leiden, Department of Data Theory, 1985.
6 Gifi A: Nonlinear Multivariate Analysis. New York, Wiley, 1990.
7 Angermeyer MC, Matschinger H: Public attitude towards psychiatric treatment. Acta Psychiatr Scand 1996;94:326–336.

Prof. M.C. Angermeyer, University of Leipzig, Department of Psychiatry,
Johannisallee 20, D–04317 Leipzig (Germany)
Tel. +49 341 972 4530, Fax +49 341 972 4539

Guimón J, Fischer W, Sartorius N (eds): The Image of Madness. The Public Facing Mental Illness and Psychiatric Treatment. Basel, Karger, 1999, pp 162–186

Determining Factors and the Effects of Attitudes towards Psychotropic Medication

W. Fischer, D. Goerg, E. Zbinden, J. Guimón

Department of Psychiatry, University Hospital, Geneva, Switzerland

In contrast to attitudes towards mental illness (which have been the object of extensive research), the general public's attitudes towards psychiatric treatment, in particular psychotropic drugs, have been the subject of little scrutiny. Only four research studies have, to our knowledge, been carried out. There was a first early study by Manheimer et al. [1]. Out of the multiple aspects tackled by this research among a sample of the general public, we shall here only examine attitudes and popular beliefs about neuroleptics. The great majority of subjects (89%) were familiar with neuroleptics and attributed to them effective calming and relaxing properties (74%). However, this positive attitude was largely counterbalanced by more reserved or even critical attitudes: 87% of the subjects interviewed considered that it was better to show willpower to solve one's own problems than take tranquilizers; others (40%) went as far as thinking that consuming drugs was a sign of personal weakness; 73% pointed to serious side effects; 80% feared harmful long-term physical effects and 69% thought that neuroleptics not only fail to heal, but cover up and hide real problems. These negative attitudes have for the authors a significant correlation with attitudes of stoicism and traditionalism. A more unfavorable attitude was observed in those subjects who considered that one of the principal causes of mental illness was a lack of moral rigor or willpower. However, the consumption of psychotropic drugs was viewed as legitimate since they were thought to be able to cure moderate or serious functioning deficits – due to depression or to anxiety – whether within the family or at work. Finally, the attitude towards tranquilizers was more favorable when the subjects themselves had had personal experience with these drugs as patients.

In a second study carried out by Guimón et al. [2, 3] among 900 patients of general practitioners by in the Basque region of Spain, the factor analysis of a scale of attitudes towards psychotropic drugs made possible the extraction of five factors: (1) attitudes based on the negative effects of psychotropic agents (stiffness, personality changes, hallucinations, loss of contact with reality (38.9% variance), (2) attitudes favoring the use of natural products for treating psychological problems (18% variance), (3) attitudes which incriminate the socio-economic system as being the cause or the motive behind the use of psychotropic drugs (12% variance), (4) attitudes which accuse psychotropic drugs of harmful sexual and reproductive aftereffects (12% variance) and (5) attitudes which touch on undesirable side effects while conceding their necessity in extreme cases (9% variance). Women expressed more reservations than men about the use of psychotropic drugs except in extreme cases. Negative attitudes increased with age and older people clearly favored natural remedies. The reverse relation was noted with regard to social status: the higher the status, the lower the expression of fear about psychotropic drugs. Generally, the fact of people consuming any type of psychoactive substances (drugs, alcohol) had a negative correlation with the attitudes towards psychotropic drugs. In addition, conservative persons were far more reserved when it came to the use of psychotropic drugs. Finally, subjects who presented more serious mental pathologies favored psychotropic drugs more and were less fearful of negative side effects.

Thirdly, the study of Angermeyer et al. [4–6] was centered on attitudes towards psychotropic drugs in general. Out of the six treatment options for each of three psychiatric diagnoses (schizophrenia, major depression and panic attacks), more than half of the subjects interviewed favored psychotherapy. Only 14% suggested pharmacotherapy. Treatment with drugs was largely out-ranked not only by psychotherapy but also by relaxation techniques (almost 50%), by natural means and remedies (a little more than 25%) and by meditation or yoga. The number of persons opposing psychotropic drugs was twice as high (41%) as those who favored them (22%) for schizophrenia and panic attacks. The opposition to medication was even greater in the case of major depression. As for diagnoses, subjects did not seem to differentiate between the various psychotropic groups and their indications. Attitudes were practically the same whether neuroleptics, antidepressants or anxiolytics were concerned. On the whole, undesirable side effects constituted the principal argument against pharmacotherapy followed by the dangers of dependency and the fact that these drugs act purely on symptoms. The results of this study confirmed those obtained by Manheimer et al. [1] regarding tranquilizers: indeed, the public considers that psychotropic prescriptions do not constitute, in and of themselves, a complete treatment for psychiatric disorders. At most, they are considered a temporary measure, a palliative while waiting for another type of treatment or in combination with a psychotherapeutic approach.

The results obtained by Benkert et al. [7] extensively corroborated those just mentioned. Whereas the vast majority of subjects interviewed agreed with the use of drugs in cases of somatic illness, only a small minority championed recourse to psychotropic drugs for patients with mental illnesses. Persons who had themselves consumed psychotropic medication were more favorable than others towards their use for depression, panic attacks as well as for obsessive-compulsive disorders. However, in this study no difference was observed in relation to schizophrenia and for other diagnoses. These authors also pointed out that the image of mental illness was stigmatized by the social marginalization associated with it. Less than one fifth of the persons interviewed would talk openly to neighbors, colleagues or acquaintances if a family member suffered from mental illness, and more than one third would never mention it. This last attitude is exceptional when a family member suffers from a physical illness.

Numerous studies have been carried out on the crucial problem of noncompliance with medication in general and psychotropic drugs in particular, giving evidence of the extent of the phenomenon and the principal variables associated with it: degree of public information about medication, its utility and the ways in which it acts, therapeutic alliance, optimum dosage in order to limit possible side effects. The importance of social and professional factors has also been studied. However, few studies have brought up the question of compliance in relation to attitudes towards medication.

In a pragmatic article, DiMatteo et al. [8] postulated that noncompliance has to be considered not as an irrational act, but rather as a rational choice that, taking into consideration the results of many studies on the subject, was based on two main factors: on the one hand, the little faith the patient had in the effectiveness of the drug, and the fact that its probable benefits might not outweigh the risks and disadvantages which its regular intake implied, on the other hand, the barriers and the difficulties perceived in observing a prescription (for example, incompatibility with daily activities) as well as the lack of family and social support for the patient. Similar conclusions were made in the studies by Lorenc and Branthwaite et al. [9] and Donovan and Blake [10].

According to the study of Angermeyer and Matschinger [11], compliance was greater when subjects considered therapies to be effective and promising. When the subjects had doubts about the efficacy of the medication they were less compliant. In these cases, subjects generally questioned the psychiatric knowledge on the etiology of the illness being treated, on the prognosis and on the therapies considered necessary by the physician. The poor compliance of patients and their social environment constituted a quasiunavoidable consequence.

Our objective in this article is to answer the following questions: what attitudes do the general public display towards different psychiatric treatments and, especially, towards psychotropic drugs? And what are the attitudes with respect to drugs in general? Which arguments are found in the public to favor or, on the contrary, to disallow different psychiatric treatments? Is there a relationship between these attitudes and the images of mental illness, between these attitudes and the therapeutic options chosen for psychiatric problems or cases of social deviancy? Which factors influence these attitudes and what are the relationships between them and subject compliance with medication?

Methods

The results presented herein are part of a study carried out among a representative sample made up of quotas (gender, age, professional activity) out of the population resident in Geneva, aged between 20 and 75. The 324 subjects thus selected answered a standardized questionnaire. Among the data gathered, we were particularly interested in the following aspects: attitudes towards psychotropic medication surveyed by means of the scale created by Guimón et al. [2], and attitudes towards medication in general evaluated on the scale of Angermeyer et al. [4]. Attitudes towards mental illness were measured with the scale of Struening and Cohen [12] and ideas about the etiology of psychiatric disorders were evaluated using a series of statements prepared by Angermeyer and Matschinger [13]. A number of social, professional, cultural and familial variables was retained.

Attitudes towards Psychotropic Drugs and Medication in General
Factor analyses were carried out for responses on the scale of attitudes towards psychotropic drugs (total variance of the 4 factors retained: 61.6%) and for the data gathered through the use of the scale of attitudes towards medication in general (total variance for 4 factors: 65.5%). The global index of attitudes towards medication – which will be used in the following analysis – was established by adding scores obtained from the four attitudinal dimensions on psychotropic medication ('negative side effects in general', 'preference for natural remedies', 'societal responsibility' and 'harmful effects on sexuality or reproduction') as well as the scores for two dimensions of the scale of attitudes on medication in general ('dangers from the consumption of medication' and 'moral judgment'). The scores used were: 1 'in total disagreement', 2 'disagree', 3 'unsure, but tend to disagree', 4 'unsure, but tend to agree', 5 'agree', 6 'in complete agreement'. In this article, the index of attitudes towards medication will be used in the form of a regrouping of the five following categories: very negative, negative, indecisive, positive, very positive. The cutoff point was at the 20th percentile.

The pertinence of this index is attested to by the fact that the four factors of the first scale and the two factors of the second correlate strongly: alpha = 0.685. As the global index refers principally to attitudes towards the use of medication in the case of psychiatric problems, we shall call this index 'attitudes towards psychotropic drugs'.

Attitudes towards Cases Presented in the Form of Vignettes and of Scenarios of Situations of Deviant Behavior in Daily Life

Another aspect of attitudes towards psychotropic drugs was drawn from answers subjects gave on three clinical vignettes and on scenarios of situations of deviant behavior in daily life. These clinical vignettes dealt with the following disorders: schizophrenia, major depression and panic attacks. The situations of deviant behavior concerned four types of conduct described in both private and public settings: withdrawal, bizarre behavior, agitation and violence. Suggestions for possible forms of medical or psychiatric treatment – or other types of assistance – were proposed.

Arguments in Support of a Refusal of Medication

The arguments against the use of medication for psychiatric disorders (which were presented in the form of vignettes) were elaborated through open-ended questions. The answers were classified into the five following categories: harmful side effects and risks of dependency, effectiveness which is dubious or which acts principally on symptoms, absence of any indication for the patient described, declarations that the patient is either not or insufficiently ill and negative positions taken with regard to all medication.

Attitudes towards Mental Illness and the Etiology of Psychiatric Disorders

We applied the scale of Struening and Cohen [12] under different conditions. Only statements which discriminated most between the two uses of the scale in preceding studies [2, 12], and for which we had detailed factorial result analyses, were retained. For each of the 5 factors which are usually found in different studies at an international level (authoritarianism, benevolence, mental hygiene ideology, social restrictiveness, family and personal responsibility, called elsewhere interpersonal etiology), as well as the new factor (community aspects) introduced in the Spanish study [2], a certain number of statements were chosen which clearly belonged to one of these factors. Fifty-eight items were thus retained in this short version of the scale. The added indices were built on the 6 factors usually mentioned in the different studies undertaken in this area. In the presentation of our results, we considered that the subjects could be deemed to have the attitudes mentioned (for example, to be authoritarian, socially restrictive) when their scores were above the 60th percentile.

In order to determine the origins of psychiatric disorders in the opinion of the subjects questioned, 18 statements were submitted to them to which they had to answer on a three-level scale: yes = 2, perhaps = 1, no = 0. The possible causes were related to the six following etiological aspects: biological (diseases of the brain, heredity), psychological (personal psychological problems, lack of willpower), psychosocial stresses (important events, difficulties in the workplace, family problems), factors linked to socialization (separation of parents during childhood, overly protective parents), societal factors (social inequality, loss of traditions and values) and the supernatural (the will of God, witchcraft, astrology).

Results

Attitudes towards Medication and Other Attitudes, Opinions and Representations

Strong Opposition to Psychotropic Medication. Our results in relation with the different aspects of psychotropic drugs indicate that public opinion is

Table 1. Percentage of subjects who agree with the declarations on the scale of attitudes towards psychotropic drugs

	%
Medication for psychiatric problems diminishes reflexes	92.0
They cause lethargy or drowsiness	90.6
Current lifestyles favor the consumption of these drugs	88.6
They act on the central nervous system and endanger the fetus	88.3
They cause passiveness and lack of initiative	87.8
They are habit-forming	86.8
Their prolonged use brings about a loss of contact with reality	84.2
The use of this medication is encouraged by a consumer-driven economy	83.8
Society favors the consumption of these drugs	82.3
These drugs diminish desire and sexual pleasure	79.4
They can cause hallucinations	73.1
As they cause personality changes, natural remedies are better	73.0
These drugs suppress personality	71.7
They cause rigidity and immobility	68.9
Natural remedies are better, neither habit-forming nor addictive	68.1
Natural remedies are not harmful for the body, therefore better	68.1
These drugs cause sexual impotence	66.2
Natural remedies can also be addictive	45.5
Drugs are more effective than natural remedies	27.3
These drugs are only harmful for pregnant women	23.5

strongly divided and, in the majority, negative with regard to these drugs. These critical – even hostile – attitudes were based on perceptions of their real – or presumed – effects.

If we add together the three answers in which subjects gave more or less formal agreement (agree totally, agree, unsure but tend to agree), it can be noted (see table 1) that more than 80% of the subjects referred to harmful effects on the central nervous system (endangering the fetus, decreasing reflexes) and on motor or psychological functioning (lethargy or drowsiness, passiveness, lack of initiative, loss of contact with reality). They criticized, in the same proportion, the addiction and dependency created by psychotropic drugs and society itself which promoted their use. Between two thirds and three fourths of the subjects interviewed also pointed out the effects on personality (changes or suppression of personality, hallucinations) as well as on the body as a whole (rigidity and immobility) and on sexuality.

Opinions in favor of natural remedies clearly formed an alternative to psychotropic drugs. According to public opinion, natural remedies possess qualities which are in opposition to psychotropic medication – and are there-

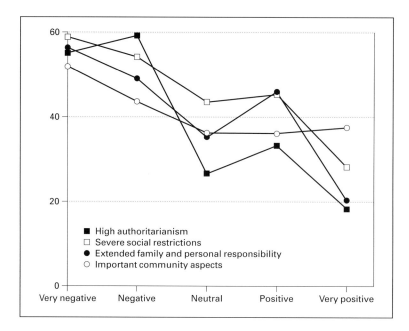

Fig. 1. Percentages of subjects beyond the 60th percentile of attitude indices towards mental illness according to attitudes towards psychotropic medication. Significance: >60th percentile on the index/≤60th percentile according to attitudes towards psychotropic medication. Authoritarianism: gamma = –0.406, p < 0.001; social restrictions: gamma = –0.270, p < 0.01; family and personal responsibility: gamma = –0.308, p < 0.001; community aspects: gamma = –0.198, p < 0.05.

fore viewed in a positive light. More than two thirds of the subjects did not think that natural remedies change the personality; they were not considered to be physically harmful, nor were they considered to be habit-forming or addictive. This alternative position was reinforced by the fact that only a little more than one fourth of subjects considered psychotropics to be more effective than natural remedies. However, almost one half found that natural remedies could also be addictive.

Attitudes towards Psychotropic Medication and Mental Illness. Is the degree to which subjects accept – or to the contrary reject – psychotropic drugs ruled by its own logic? Or are attitudes towards medication – positive or negative – linked to other attitudes, other opinions? If so, do these different attitudes and opinions constitute a specific system of representation?

First of all, with regard to attitudes towards mental illness and psychiatric patients, a very significant covariation existed with attitudes towards medication (see fig. 1). The group of subjects with very negative attitudes towards medication included, in the majority, people with pronounced authoritarian traits (55%). Stating categorically that psychiatric patients were completely different from other patients, these subjects favored a strict differentiation between mental patients and those suffering from a somatic illness. They also said that psychiatric patients could easily be distinguished from other people, their distinctive trait being a lack of willpower or moral fiber.

Those persons with the most negative opinions on psychotropic medication were also those who would place the greatest social restrictions on psychiatric patients, even to the point of creating barriers of segregation: 59.2% held very rigid opinions on this subject. They thought that the children of the mentally ill should not be allowed to visit their parents in hospital, that patients should be sterilized and that mental illness left indelible traces, even when patients considered themselves to be cured.

It might appear surprising that the most radical opponents of psychotropic drugs also blamed the family or the patient for the mental illness. It was the case for 56.4% of this group, whereas only one fifth of persons who were more favorably inclined towards psychotropic medication shared this opinion. Thus, the adversaries of psychiatric pharmacotherapy were most often in agreement with statements according to which 'many people become mentally ill to avoid difficulties in daily life', that patients had parents who 'were not very interested in them' or who separated or divorced very early in their lives. They also thought that mental illness could be transmitted – like a communicable disease – by adults to children. This group appeared to assume that an upbringing provided by a mentally ill adult would necessarily produce psychiatric disorders in any children they might foster.

In analogy to authoritarianism and favoring social barriers was the endorsement of the idea that the family or the patient was to blame for mental illness. The criticism these subjects expressed took the form, above all, of a condemnation of a supposed lack of morality and a deterioration in society today: the disintegration of the family, the refusal to take responsibility.

As shown in figure 1, attitudes towards mental illness changed in a highly significant fashion when attitudes towards psychotropic drugs became more positive. Whether authoritarianism, social restrictions or family and personal responsibility were concerned, the percentage of the most fervent proponents diminished drastically. Thus, among subjects with very positive attitudes towards psychotropic drugs, only 18.3% adopted a very authoritarian attitude towards patients, 28.3% would enact severe social restrictions and only 20.4% believed the patient and his or her family were responsible for the illness.

We found almost the same tendency when analyzing the responses to the possible causes of the psychiatric disorders presented in the vignettes.

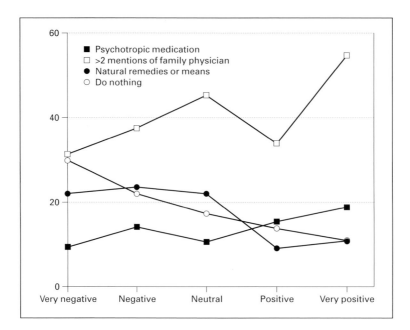

Fig. 2. Percentages of mentions of different forms of advice on confronting situations of deviant behavior in daily life according to attitudes towards psychotropic medication. Significance: mention/no mention of proposed advice according to attitudes towards psychotropic medication. Psychotropic medication: gamma $= 0.169$, nonsignificant; > 2 family physicians: gamma $= 0.177$, $p < 0.01$; natural remedies or means: gamma $= -0.249$, $p < 0.05$; do nothing: gamma $= -0.297$, $p < 0.01$.

The most categorical opponents of psychotropic drugs significantly more frequently mentioned psychosocial (important life events, difficulties in the workplace, within the family, with the partner) and psychological factors (overprotective parents, personal psychological problems, lack of will-power) than those persons expressing more positive views on psychotropic medication.

Attitudes towards Psychotropic Medication and Advice on Confronting Situations of Deviant Behavior in Daily Life. The analysis of responses given by subjects on how to deal with situations of deviant behavior in daily life also revealed significant differences in respect to attitudes about psychotropic drugs (see fig. 2). In particular, as expected, a direct correlation (close to a level of significance) existed between attitudes towards medication and the option to take psychotropic medication. We also noted a direct correlation between these attitudes and the frequent allusion (3 times and more) 'to go see the doctor'. Less than one third of those decisively opposed to psychotropic medication suggested consulting the family physician, whereas more than half (54.7%) of those having the highest opinion of psychotropic drugs did. We, therefore, noted a very clear tendency among opponents of medication to neither consult a physician specialized in somatic illness nor a psychiatrist when faced with situations of deviant behavior. This was confirmed by two other results: opponents, in great numbers, preferred natural remedies or means (nearly one fourth), whereas this opinion was only held by about a tenth of those in favor of psychotropic medication. In addition, almost one third of those showing very negative attitudes thought that nothing should be done in such situations, i.e. 3 times more than for those with very positive attitudes towards psychotropic drugs.

Attitudes towards Psychotropic Medication and Therapeutic Approaches in Cases Presented in the Form of Clinical Vignettes. The results of the therapeutic proposals which were considered to be most useful in the psychiatric cases presented by vignettes confirmed the answers given for situations of deviant behavior, which made little reference to psychopathological characteristics. The most positive attitudes towards psychotropic drugs corresponded to specific psychiatric options: 4 out of 10 people suggested recourse to them and almost two thirds to individual psychotherapy (see fig. 3). In contrast, only 3% of the most categorical opponents proposed psychotropic medication and slightly more than 40% individual psychotherapy. These proportions rose at the rate at which attitudes towards psychotropic drugs became more positive. In an entirely coherent fashion, reservations expressed about psychotherapy and the refusal to endorse the use of psychotropic medication operated to the advantage of other methods considered to be less intrusive or alternative. In fact, between one fifth and one fourth of the opponents to psychotropic medication preferred recourse to relaxation techniques, to natural remedies or to the practice of meditation or yoga. These approaches were only supported by one tenth of subjects with more positive attitudes.

Reasons for Refusing Psychotropic Medication. Questioned on why they did not consider the use of psychotropic drugs as a possible therapeutic solution for the cases presented in the form of vignettes, subjects with very negative attitudes towards psychotropic drugs mentioned their negative attitude towards medication in general and, secondly, undesirable or even harmful side effects (see fig. 4). More than one third brought up the latter. Approximately one fourth thought that the efficacy of psychotropic medication was debatable because it only acts on symptoms and is, at best, a temporary solution. And a further one fourth even doubted that the person described was really ill, or they believed the person had a problem which was primarily psychological in nature. According to these subjects, medication was not advisable in such cases. The proportion of subjects who argued in favor of a refusal to use

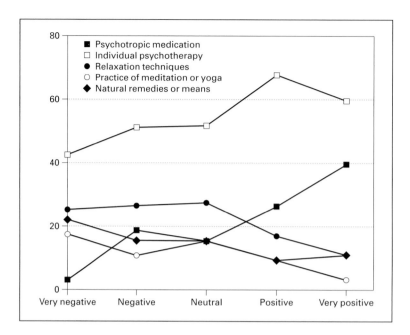

Fig. 3. Percentages of therapeutic proposals in cases presented in the clinical vignettes according to attitudes towards psychotropic medication. Significance: mention of the therapeutic proposal/no mention according to attitudes towards psychotropic medication. Psychotropic medication: gamma = 0.476, p < 0.01; individual psychotherapy: gamma = 0.205, p < 0.01; relaxation techniques: gamma = –0.220, p < 0.05; practice of meditation or yoga: gamma = –0.296, p < 0.05; natural remedies or means: gamma = –0.224, p < 0.05.

psychotropic drugs for one of the four reasons indicated decreased progressively with a better acceptance of psychotropic medication. Among those subjects with very positive attitudes, only about one tenth mentioned reasons for refusal.

Therefore, we observed that positive or negative attitudes regarding psychotropic drugs were interconnected with the subjects' other opinions and representations. The results obtained allow us to sketch the following portraits. The most fervent champions of psychotropic drugs agreed in saying that both the cases presented in situations in daily life, and those described in the vignettes were characterized by undeniable psychiatric aspects. In this regard, they required a particular medical-psychiatric approach in the form of individual psychotherapy or treatment by medication. Alternative or less intrusive methods would, therefore, be ineffective and inoperable. Side effects, deemed to be minor in this context, constituted in some ways the price that must be paid to guarantee the efficacy of psychotropic medication. Defining the person

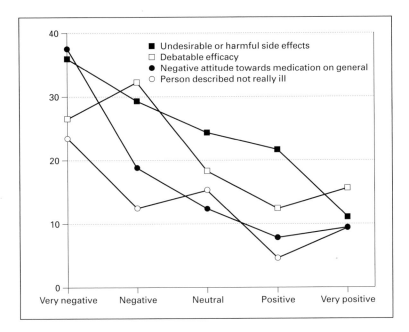

Fig. 4. Percentages of mentions of reasons for refusing psychotropic medication according to attitudes towards psychotropic medication. Significance: mention of the reasons/no mention according to attitudes towards psychotropic medication. Undesirable or harmful side effects: gamma = –0.308, p < 0.001; debatable efficacy: gamma = –0.250, p < 0.01; negative attitudes towards medication in general; gamma = –0.463, p < 0.001; person described not really ill: gamma = –0.313, p < 0.01.

in the cases described as mentally ill, those with a very positive attitude towards psychotropic drugs also displayed more tolerant views on psychiatry and mental illness. They expressed, in particular, more open-mindedness and more nuanced opinions than others: they abstained from making moral judgments about psychiatric patients and rarely suggested imposing social restrictions or segregation.

The opposite pole of opinion which was most negative towards psychotropic medication was paired with a tendency to deny, or at least not to recognize, the psychiatric conditions and aspects of the persons and situations presented. The subjects who shared this position stated most frequently that the persons described were not ill and so, consequently, nothing should be done. Their disavowal of psychotropic drugs, and their reticence about referring such people to a physician, a psychiatrist or a psychologist appeared as two facets of a more generalized opposition to medicine itself as well as to psychiatry. By considering psychiatric patients as persons who are different in many

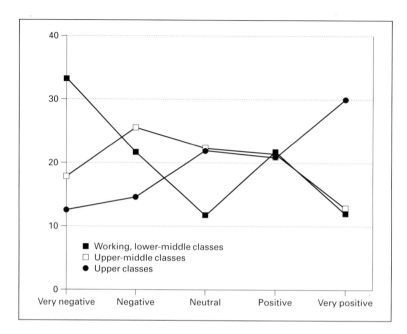

Fig. 5. Distribution (%) of attitudes towards psychotropic medication according to the social status of the subjects. Significance: gamma = 0.280, p < 0.01.

ways, they promoted a very authoritarian view, basing their judgments on moral bias. They would impose on psychiatric patients not only segregation, but restrictions on their rights and prerogatives that any citizen might normally exercise without interference.

Factors Determining Attitudes towards Psychotropic Medication
Structural and Cultural Influences on Attitudes. No sociodemographic characteristic was significantly associated with attitudes towards medication in general and psychotropic drugs in particular: neither age nor gender nor marital status nor family situation. In contrast, these attitudes varied greatly with the social status of the subjects. As figure 5 shows, positive attitudes were much more prevalent in the upper-middle and upper classes: persons holding managerial positions, technicians, teachers, the liberal professions. More than half had either positive (20.8%), or very positive (30.2%) attitudes; approximately one fifth (21.9%) were neutral and slightly more than one fourth had negative (12.5%) or very negative (14.6%) opinions. Among the working class, this negative polarity covered 55% of subjects, 11.7% were neutral, while only one third (33.3%) defined themselves as having positive or very positive attitudes towards psychotropic

medication. Lower-middle class subjects occupied an intermediate position, slightly closer to working class values than to those of the upper-middle or upper class. These attitude differences according to social status were confirmed by the statistically significant correlation ($p < 0.05$) between income and the attitude scale towards psychotropic drugs. Subjects with a lower income displayed a marked tendency towards more negative attitudes; these diminished clearly the more the income of the subject rose.

A second factor which influenced attitudes in a significant manner was of a cultural nature. These attitudes were positively and strongly correlated to several indicators of the sociocultural level of subjects: the higher this level was, the more positive were the attitudes ($p < 0.001$). Thus, 56.3% of university graduates showed positive or very positive attitudes, but this was the case for only 36.6% of those without higher education. Forty-four percent of the latter were rather hostile or even very hostile to psychotropic medication as against only 23.5% of university graduates. Subjects with studies ranging in the intermediate level described themselves, from the point of view of their attitudes towards psychotropic drugs, as also being at an intermediate level.

The same differences appeared when we took into account the type of professional training ($p < 0.001$). It was interesting to note that attitudes towards psychotropic drugs even seemed to be influenced by transgenerational cultural factors since the same significant variations stood out for both the father's ($p < 0.01$) and the mother's ($p < 0.05$) educational levels.

Fields of Specific Activities, Participation in Volunteer Organizations and Ideological Commitments. We also inquired into the possibility that certain types of activity had an influence over attitudes towards psychotropic medication. There were activities which appeared to put subjects and/or their families into professional contact with humanitarian endeavors in society, such as working in the medical field, in the field of psychiatry or mental handicap, in the social, socioeducational and teaching sectors. Those among the interviewees who belonged in this category showed significantly more positive attitudes ($p < 0.05$) than those who did not have such professional interaction. The same thing applied to social or ideological commitments. Subjects showed more clearly positive attitudes ($p < 0.001$) when they were involved in volunteer organizations or associations in one of the above-mentioned fields, or pursued humanitarian or ecological concerns. Thus, 56.4% of those who were members of at least one group presented positive or very positive attitudes towards psychotropic drugs and 24.3% negative or even very negative attitudes. The corresponding proportions were of 34.6 and 44.7% in subjects who were not active in any sort of humanitarian endeavor.

Proximity to Psychiatry. Living or working close to a residential or outpatient unit for psychiatric patients had no influence on attitudes towards

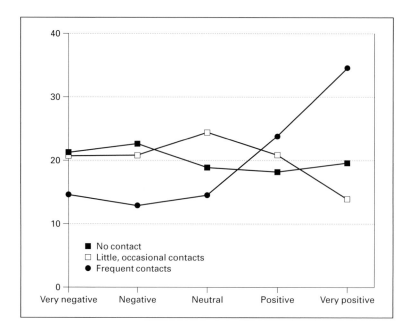

Fig. 6. Distribution (%) of attitudes towards psychotropic medication according to the frequency of contact with persons with mental problems. Significance: gamma = 0.138, p < 0.05.

psychotropic drugs. In contrast, what could be called relational proximity (to be familiar with such institutions as a volunteer, for professional reasons or as a visitor) caused markedly more positive attitudes (p < 0.001). More than half of subjects (54.5%) with the closest links to psychiatry had positive or very positive attitudes as against only slightly more than one third who had only distant connections to this field. The proportion of negative or very negative attitudes amounted to 28.8% among the former and 45.5% among the latter.

Contact with Individuals Having Suffered from Psychological or Psychiatric Problems and the Subject's Own Personal Experience. Contact with relatives, friends, colleagues or acquaintances having experienced psychological or psychiatric problems also contributed to fashioning positive attitudes towards psychotropic drugs: the more frequent the contact, or the more serious the problem in question, the more positive were the subject's attitudes (p < 0.05, see fig. 6). But it must be pointed out that the impact of this contact, while statistically significant, was less decisive than the subject's relational proximity and social or ideological commitments. In effect, we observed positive or very positive attitudes among more than half (58.1%) of the subjects who had more frequent contacts with persons with mental problems and a little more than one fourth of these (27.2%) were hostile to psychotropic drugs. The latter view was shared by 43.5% of subjects having little or no contact, while 37.7% held positive attitudes. We therefore noted that a higher frequency of contact was a prerequisite for positive attitudes; there was little difference between occasional contacts and none in influencing attitudes.

Personal experience with mental problems created similar differences. Such a personal experience was associated with positive views in half of the subjects (49.4%) and with a negative outlook in almost one third (32.0%). Among subjects who had never been personally confronted by such problems, we noted there was a proportion of positive attitudes of 36.6% and negative ones amounting to 42.4%.

Attitudes in Respect to Psychotropic Medication, the Viewpoints of the Patient's Entourage on Medication and Compliance

Not only the attitudes but also the representations of mental illness by opponents and protagonists were reinforced by the views held by their families, friends and acquaintances. The answers to questions concerning whether members of the subject's entourage were systematically opposed to medication showed a very strong correlation with the attitudes of subjects themselves towards psychotropic drugs (p < 0.001). Subjects who lived with persons who were opposed to medication had, in the majority (53.4%), negative or very negative attitudes and only slightly more than one fourth (28.7%) expressed a positive view on psychotropic drugs. In contrast, almost half (44.9%) of subjects who did not know anyone who was systematically opposed to medication had favorable opinions and a third expressed a negative perspective.

The most striking effects of attitudes towards psychotropic drugs could be found at the level of compliance with pharmaceutical treatment in general. Compliance was first measured through questions inquiring into whether the subject thought it advisable to take only some of the drugs prescribed by a physician, to decrease dosage or to stop it entirely without seeking the physician's advice. The index of compliance assembled from responses to these questions showed that slightly more than one third of the interviewees favored a high level of compliance, one fourth an intermediate level of compliance, one sixth a low level of compliance and approximately one fifth a very low level of compliance. We observed an important covariation between this index and attitudes (see fig. 7). While limiting this study to giving evidence on results of extreme positions, we noted that only one fifth (21.9%) of subjects characterized by very negative attitudes admitted to total compliance with medical prescriptions. Almost half of this group (46.9%) ranked at a very high

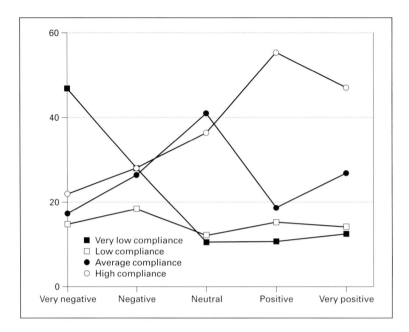

Fig. 7. Distribution (%) of compliance with medical prescriptions according to attitudes towards psychotropic medication. Significance: gamma = 0.324, p < 0.001.

level of noncompliance. Inversely, almost half of subjects with very positive attitudes were also among those with the highest level of compliance and only one eighth (12.5%) had a very low level of compliance. In a rather surprising way, the proportion of strongly or very strongly compliant subjects was as high among the subjects having neutral attitudes as those characterized by very positive attitudes. The positive attitudes included two clearly opposed groups: the strongly compliant and the others who were represented here in almost equal proportions.

A second measure of compliance concerned the reactions of subjects to cases where a prescribed medication caused undesirable side effects: a decrease in dosage decided on by the subject him- or herself, immediately stopping the prescribed medication or replacing it with another with which the subject has had personal experience and knows that it causes no side effects. This second type of compliance was better than the former since more than half of the subjects (57.7%) ranked at a high level of compliance, one fourth at an intermediate level and one sixth only at a low level. There again, a high correlation (see fig. 8) was found. In the case of positive attitudes, almost three quarters of subjects (71.9%) remained totally compliant even if side effects occurred

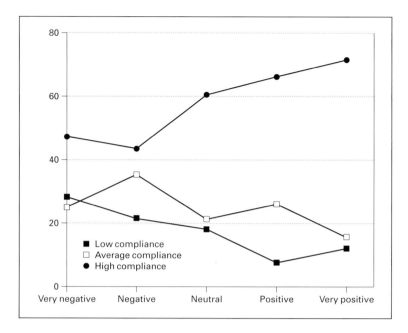

Fig. 8. Distribution (%) of compliance with medication presenting undesirable side effects according to attitudes towards psychotropic medication. Significance: gamma = 0.275, p < 0.001.

and only 1 out of 8 showed a low level of compliance. Adversely, less than half of those who had negative or very negative attitudes had a high level of compliance, with an intermediate and a low level of compliance each amounting to one fourth. We encountered a clear differentiation between those subjects with a high level of compliance and those at an intermediate or at a low level of compliance. The size of these two groups decreased in an almost linear fashion as we progressed from the very negative pole of attitudes towards psychotropic drugs to its positive opposite.

Discussion

Opinions on Psychotropic Drugs

The public generally showed very negative opinions about psychotropic drugs. The vast majority of statements, containing critical or even negative judgments, were approved by more than two thirds of subjects interviewed. Despite the difference in generation and in culture, the results Manheimer et al. [1] obtained in 1973 in the United States were very similar to ours.

Whether the question asked concerned lethargy or drowsiness, loss of contact with reality, physical damage after long periods of drug use or addiction or dependency, these authors obtained unfavorable opinions on neuroleptics in the same proportions as those we got in Geneva for psychotropic drugs in general. The subjects endorsed what Klerman [quoted in 1] called 'pharmacological Calvinism', suggesting that strong currents of conservatism also exist with regard to the moral issue of recourse to psychotropic medication.

The study of Benkert et al. [7], carried out in Germany, also revealed that these attitudes were, to a large degree, still prevalent: psychotropic drugs were perceived by two thirds (66%) of the population as having more negative side effects than advantages and only one seventh (15%) considered them to have more positive than negative aspects. The subjects judged the following side effects particularly unacceptable (which supports our own results): sexual difficulties such as impotence, dependency and addiction, motor function problems, rigidity or lack of mobility, hallucinations and loss of contact with reality. These different negative side effects were mentioned by more than three quarters of subjects in our study and provoked the strongest reservations in those interviewed by Benkert et al. [7].

The condemnation of side effects in general and, in particular, the important risks of addiction to psychotropic drugs seemed to inspire the most virulent fears. In addition, Angermeyer et al. [4] pointed out that subjects interviewed advanced a third argument: the effectiveness of psychopharmacological therapy was dubious and debatable. They considered that psychotropic drugs merely transfer, or even exacerbate, problems rather than solving them. Subjects think that, because these drugs act only on symptoms, the very nature of the help they provide in calming patients is ephemeral. Under these conditions, psychotropic drugs would only be a second or last therapeutic choice. Our study also confirmed these results.

Opposition to Psychotropic Drugs as a Symbol for Adversaries of Medicine and Psychiatry

The work of Angermeyer et al. [4, 6] showed that the proportion of the public who refused psychopharmacology was, on the contrary, much more favorably inclined towards other treatment, especially psychotherapy whether or not this included the prescription of psychotropic drugs. In summary, there were two public schools of thought which endorsed either biological psychiatry or classical psychotherapy; a third school championed alternative psychiatric-type solutions (such as relaxation) or favored alternative concepts (meditation, yoga, natural remedies, acupuncture).

Through the use of methodology which resembled that in the work quoted above (questions about therapeutic solutions to the clinical cases presented in the vignettes), we obtained results which were considerably different. Recourse to psychotropic drugs did not appear to contravene psychotherapy. Subjects with the most negative attitudes towards medication suggested, in response to the clinical situations presented, significantly less frequently either drugs or psychotherapy. The more positive the subject's attitudes towards psychotropic drugs, the greater the tendency to opt for either of the two psychiatric treatments to the detriment of nonmedical solutions: natural remedies, meditation, yoga and relaxation. As the adversaries of psychotropic drugs were less willing to advise the use of the two specifically psychiatric forms of therapy, does this mean that they adopted the same critical and removed attitudes towards psychiatry and medicine in general that they do towards psychotropic medication? If this is the case, we are faced with a more general orientation which influences, in a restricting or even negative way, subjects' attitudes not only towards psychotropic medication, but towards medicine and psychiatry.

Several results support our interpretation. Opposition to psychotropic drugs most often came from those subjects who maintained that the persons described in the vignettes were not ill. As the subjects did not take illness into account, a psychiatric approach was, therefore, unnecessary, whatever the type of treatment foreseen. Or the subjects considered the problems to be psychological in nature and that drug therapy was not indicated. Responses to situations of deviant behavior in daily life conformed to the same logic. There again, the option 'to do nothing' was most frequently made by adversaries of psychotropic medication who also less frequently chose the option of intervention by a psychiatrist or a somatic physician.

More fundamentally, this distant attitude with regard to medicine in general and to psychiatry and its medication in particular can be interpreted in terms of class differences such as those described by Hoggart [14] with reference to the working class. An interesting analogy can be made here for several observations emanating from our study. Firstly, subjects opposing recourse to psychotropic drugs, to medicine and psychiatry in the different situations presented during the interview were mainly recruited among blue- or white-collar workers, among those with a relatively low level of education and professional training and whose parents had also figured at the bottom of the professional ladder in terms of qualification and, finally, among the most financially disadvantaged social groups. These results resembled those analyzed by Kadushin [15] and Goerg et al. [16] when they attributed importance, with regard to access to psychiatry, to what Kadushin called the 'friends and supporters of psychotherapy'. In contrast to members of the working class, 'these proponents tend to contact directly the most prestigious institutions, presenting problems which have affinities with psychoanalytical or psychodynamic approaches for the cases involved' [16]. These studies confirmed that proximity to psychiatry and associated psychiatric 'sophistication' were, to a great extent, the consequence of the subject's level of education, social class and employment in certain fields of activity already mentioned here: health care systems, education and teaching. Adherence to the values of psychiatry was thus linked to social class: the members of the upper classes and, in a less noticeable way, those of the middle classes shared a belief in the values of psychiatric orientation more than the working classes did. For the working class, their skepticism resulted from a lack of belief in the value of psychiatry or from their adherence to other systems of belief when they were confronted with problems which a majority of subjects coming from other social classes would refer to psychiatry.

Franz et al. [17] arrived at similar conclusions. Their study covered patients who refused the option of psychotherapy advised by their therapists. Among the reasons motivating this refusal, 34% of patients mentioned that psychotherapy did not seem necessary either because they thought they could solve their problems without therapy, or because they considered the problems to be primarily of a somatic nature. This declaration of what the authors call 'personal autonomy' and the resulting refusal of psychiatric treatment was principally encountered in persons with a low level of education ($p < 0.05$) and among men. For the latter, other studies [18] have shown that, in contrast to women, they were much less willing to accept therapy with a psychoanalytical orientation or to define their problems at this level.

The study of the cultural mistrust of African-Americans [19] corroborated this interpretation of the distance the economically disadvantaged feel towards medicine and psychiatry. A stronger mistrust of whites was significantly associated with more negative attitudes with regard to requesting help from institutions, whose personnel is mainly white, and was linked to a fear that the services offered by white advisers might be less appropriate.

Determining Factors Influencing Attitudes towards Psychotropic Drugs

As in other studies [4, 5], the sociodemographic variables (gender, age, marital status, family situation) did not exert any influence on attitudes towards psychotropic drugs; nor did the authors of these studies note an impact from cultural or professional variables. In contrast, our study gives evidence of the very clear relationship between attitudes towards psychotropic drugs and sociocultural level: the education, professional training and degrees of the subjects interviewed. The higher social and cultural levels were systematically associated with more favorable attitudes towards psychotropic medication. The presence of an impact crossing generations (the effect of parents' cultural level) highlighted the probable influence of factors which are very deeply engrained in our culture and which prevent rapid changes in mentality with regard to the image of mental illness and the social representation of psychiatric treatment.

Support for this hypothesis can be found in the fact that 3 other factors determine important differences in attitude. They are relational proximity to psychiatry, personal experience of psychological problems or of mental disorders, and social or ideological commitment to organizations and associations working in the areas of mental illness, mental handicap, medicine, education and ecological or pacifist movements. One of the most efficient instruments to effect a change in attitudes towards psychiatry and mental illness, towards psychiatric therapy and psychotropic medication would seem, therefore, to reside in a direct encounter with affected persons and with psychiatry itself and with the services dealing with disabilities, educational, social or environmental problems, either because of personal implication, or because of an active commitment to these causes within the framework of associations or organizations.

Through the comparison of subgroups in their sample (which were assembled according to the extent of their exposure to mental illness), Angermeyer and Matschinger [11] obtained results which substantiated our own hypothesis. However, they did not study the impact of attitudes on psychotropic medication, but on mental illness. Subjects who had experience of mental illness (personally or within their family or circle of acquaintance) were characterized by more open-minded attitudes towards mental patients and by a greater inclination to interact with them. They also reacted with less fear of them and displayed less hostility and less distance. As very close statistical relationships exist between subject attitudes about mental illness itself and those towards psychotropic drugs, the results of the German study corroborated our own conclusions.

Compliance

Numerous studies have been carried out on the crucial problem of noncompliance in relation to medication in general and psychotropic drugs in particular, giving evidence of the extent of the phenomenon and the principal aspects linked to it. The importance of social and professional factors have also been analyzed. But very little research has touched on the question of compliance in relation to attitudes towards medication. In addition, in almost all the studies, compliance was defined as both a sign of total and wholehearted confidence in the physician, and as appropriate behavior in relation to illness and the therapeutic means available. Noncompliance brought into question confidence in the physician and in the efficacy of his or her treatment; it also constitutes an unacceptable waste.

The results of our study show, nevertheless, that noncompliance is not a behavior which is contrary to all logic; it cannot be considered to be a manifestation of random choices. Compliance and noncompliance appear, to the contrary, to be linked in a coherent fashion to the two following facts: firstly, attitudes in respect to medication in general and psychotropic drugs in particular and secondly, to opinions in the family and entourage with regard to the consumption of medication. Noncompliance is, in effect, justifiable behavior that can even be deemed to be necessary when the subject's attitudes and convictions and those of his or her entourage point out the possible dangers of medication. Strong compliance, in its turn, is a rational act when the subject's opinions and those of his or her entourage are motivated by principle and by adherence to the physician's code for the prescription of medication.

On the basis of results from numerous studies, DiMatteo et al. [8] postulated that noncompliance should be considered to be a rational choice based on the patient's evaluation of the ratio of presumed effectiveness and possible benefits to the risks and inconvenience that its regular consumption implies. The latter were not compensated for by the advantages taken into account. The obstacles and difficulties that may arise in observing the prescription may favor noncompliance, as does a lack of family and social support. Lorenc Branthwaite [9] and Donovan and Blake [10] reached the same conclusion.

Having studied the arguments put forward by chronic patients concerning their noncompliance with medical prescriptions, Thorne [20] underlined two principal factors which were identified among patients suffering for long periods from a chronic illness such as diabetes. Patients explained their diminished compliance with professional recommendations as the result of a choice to personally assume responsibility for their health. Having become, due to their illness, increasingly familiar with the medical world (professionals, medication) and increasingly conscious of their own singular psychological and physiological responses to the process, they had been led to question authority: who should be held accountable for decisions taken with regard to treatment? And, by taking responsibility for these decisions and for the risks to their own health, they challenge socially accepted beliefs which would give this power to professionals alone.

Heightened confidence in their own ability to decide and to assume personal responsibility for their own health, leads these patients to increasingly question the authority of professionals to be considered sole judge in these matters. They gradually acquire the conviction that professionals act in line with their own set of beliefs rather than in accordance with universal truths. Casting doubt on the arguments of these professionals, or even on their authority in the field of chronic illness, these patients begin to discuss and negotiate their own decisions. They call upon professionals to justify or abandon their status as experts, which automatically creates difficulties and conflict in the doctor-patient relationship. The distance of members of the working class – through their negative attitudes towards psychotropic drugs – in respect to psychiatry and medicine in general seems to play the same role in our study. It acts in opposition to the logic of the medical and scientific world: evoking another form of logic and other principles of evaluation and appreciation which, as was shown by Hoggart [14], tend to reject submission to 'others', i.e. to those persons who take decisions over them and who control the different spheres of their lives. Thus, the prolonged experience of chronic illness and frequent interaction with professionals of the health care system seem to neutralize the usual impact of social factors on attitudes towards medication and compliance.

References

1   Manheimer DI, Davidson ST, Balter MB, Mellinger GD, Cisin IH, Parry HJ: Popular attitudes and beliefs about tranquilizers. Am J Psychiatry 1973;130:1246–1253.
2   Guimón J, Ozamiz A, Viar I: Actitudes de la población ante el consumo terapeutico de psicofármacos. VII Reunión de la sociedad Española de Psiquiatría Biológica, Madrid, 1979, pp 165–175.
3   Guimón J, Ozamiz A, Ylla L, Echevarria A, Sanjuan C: Automedicación en población general y en pacientes médicos; in Casas M (ed): Trastornos psíquicos en las toxicomanias. Barcelona, Ediciones en neurociencias, 1992, pp 341–354.
4   Angermeyer MC, Däumer R, Matschinger H: Benefits and risks of psychotropic medication in the eyes of the general public: Results of a survey in the Federal Republic of Germany. Pharmacopsychiatry 1993;26:114–120.
5   Angermeyer MC, Held T, Görtler D: Pro und contra: Psychotherapie und Psychopharmakotherapie im Urteil der Bevölkerung. Psychother Psychosom Med Psychol 1993;43:286–292.
6   Angermeyer MC: Einstellung der Bevölkerung zu Psychopharmaka; in Naber K, Müller-Spahn F (eds): Clozapin, Pharmakologie und Klinik eines atypischen Neuroleptikums. Heidelberg, Springer, 1994, pp 113–123.
7   Benkert O, Kepplinger HM, Sobota K: Psychopharmaka im Widerstreit: Eine Studie zur Akzeptanz von Psychopharmaka – Bevölkerungsumfrage und Medienanalyse. Heidelberg, Springer, 1995.
8   DiMatteo MR, Reiter R, Gambone JC: Enhancing medication adherence through communication and informed collaborative choice. Health Commun 1994;6:253–265.
9   Lorenc L, Branthwaite A: Are older adults less compliant with prescribed medication than younger adults? Br J Clin Psychol 1993;32:485–492.
10 Donovan JL, Blake DR: Patient non-compliance: Deviance or reasoned decision-making? Soc Sci Med 1992;34:507–513.
11 Angermeyer MC, Matschinger H: The effect of personal experience with mental illness on the attitude towards individuals suffering from mental disorders. Soc Psychiatry Psychiatr Epidemiol 1996;31:321–326.
12 Struening EL, Cohen J: Factorial invariance and other psychometric characteristics of five opinions about mental illness factors. Educ Psychol Meas 1963;23:289–297.
13 Angermeyer MC, Matschinger H: Lay beliefs about schizophrenic disorder: The results of a population survey in Germany. Acta Psychiatr Scand 1994;89(suppl 382):39–45.
14 Hoggart R: La culture du pauvre. Etude sur le style de vie des classes populaires en Angleterre. Le sens commun. Paris, Editions de Minuit, 1970.
15 Kadushin C: Why People Go to Psychiatrists. New York, Atherton Press, 1969.

16 Goerg D, Zbinden E, Duvanel B: Congruence patients-thérapeutes et dropout en psychiatrie ambulatoire publique. Sci Soc Santé 1990;8:49–71.

17 Franz M, Dilo K, Schepank H, Reister G: Warum 'nein' zur Psychotherapie? Kognitive Stereotypien psychogen erkrankter Patienten aus einer Bevölkerungsstichprobe im Zusammenhang mit der Ablehnung eines Psychotherapieangebotes. Psychother Psychosom Med Psychol 1993;43:278–285.

18 Bland RC, Newman SC, Orn H: Health care utilization for emotional problems: Results from a community survey. Can J Psychiatry 1990;35:397–400.

19 Nickerson KJ, Helms JE, Terrell F: Cultural mistrust, opinions about mental illness, and black students' attitudes toward seeking psychological help from white counselors. J Couns Psychol 1994;41:378–385.

20 Thorne SE: Constructive noncompliance in chronic illness. Holistic Nurs Pract 1990;5:62–69.

Werner Fischer, Unité d'investigation sociologique, Département de Psychiatrie, Hôpitaux Universitaires de Genève, 2, chemin du Petit-Bel-Air, CH–1225 Chêne-Bourg (Switzerland)
Tel. +41 22 305 57 53, Fax +41 22 305 57 99

Guimón J, Fischer W, Sartorius N (eds): The Image of Madness. The Public Facing Mental Illness and Psychiatric Treatment. Basel, Karger, 1999, pp 187–196

....
Attitudes towards Psychotropic Medication among Medical Students

Andreas Hillert

Medizinisch-Psychosomatische Klinik Roseneck, Center for Behavioral Medicine affiliated to the Faculty of Medicine of the Ludwig Maximilians University Munich, Prien am Chiemsee, Germany

Medical Students: A Target Group of Psychiatric Attitude Research

As opposed to the general public, patients and mental health professionals, medical students scarcely have been a target group of psychiatric attitude research. The main goal of the inquiries of students has been their view of psychiatrists, of psychiatry as a clinical and scientific discipline [1–4] and psychiatry as a desired occupation [5–7]. At least in older publications a distinct inferiority complex of psychiatrists towards other medical disciplines, such as internal medicine or surgery, is evident: the basis of several investigations has been the assumption that psychiatry is negatively rated by the public, patients and students, and therefore needs further legitimization. The items used in the questionnaires often include negative stereotypes. The specific 'attitude to psychiatry scale' [3] includes items like: 'psychiatrists tend to be more emotionally unstable than other doctors' or 'within medicine, psychiatry is one of the less important specialities'. A lower degree of agreement with these statements could be interpreted to reflect an amelioration of the image of psychiatry. In these investigations the subject of psychopharmacological treatment was touched only indirectly.

Independently of the tradition of psychiatric attitude research, the illness concepts held by medical students, the extent of their consideration of psychosomatic aspects and their attitudes towards psychosomatic training have been the subject of research [8, 9]. Although biological (or somatic) illness concepts are quite popular, psychosomatic courses are rated to be of importance and helpful in medical training.

Only two studies focusing on medical students' attitudes to psycho-pharmacological treatment have been published: Linden and Becker [10] and Angermeyer et al. [11], and Hillert et al. [12]. The study of Kröber [13] also included several relevant aspects.

The Relevance of the Students' Attitudes towards Psychopharmacology

The effectiveness of psychotropic drugs in the treatment of serious psychiatric disorders like schizophrenia, mania or depression has been proven in countless studies. From the psychiatric point of view the majority of patients suffering from these disorders should receive psychotropic drugs, as no similar effective alternative treatment is known. In the clinical practice only a relatively small number of these patients really take their medication according to the prescriptions. Noncompliant behavior, often causing an insufficient therapeutic outcome, relapses and negative psychosocial consequences (the social network as well as the quality of life are at risk), is a highly complex phenomenon: the discrepancies between the pharmacological and the patients' subjective side effects have to be considered, taking the patients' individual illness concepts and their being 'inside psychosis' into consideration. Beside the patient's social network and the media [14], the consulting physician is assumed to have a lasting influence on the patients' conceptions of illness and their compliance. In the clinical practice it can be frequently observed that patient behavior is negatively biased by insufficiently informed medical professionals; at least some of their dislike of psychotropic drugs derives from antipsychiatric ideologies. After passing their examinations medical students will become medical professionals. Their perception of psychopharmacological treatment therefore will be of great therapeutic consequence.

Can individual illness concepts and attitudes towards psychotropic drugs be changed? Medical education can be taken as a model to gauge improvement in knowledge and student attitudes towards psychotropic medication. Of course, the medical student's special situation has to be taken into account when discussing the implications of the findings.

Attitudes of Medical and Psychology Students towards Psychopharmacology

In 1983, medical and psychology students at the University of Berlin answered open questions on psychopharmacological treatment [10]. To avoid negative implications [see 15], Linden and Becker [10] used the following open questions: (1) Please give reasons for and against a psychopharmacological treatment. (2) A friend is treated by his doctor with psychotropic drugs. What would be your advice? (3) What would you do, if a doctor advises you to take psychotropic drugs over a long period? The answers of 212 medical and 85 psychology students were evaluated according to a text-analytical procedure. Forty-one medical students were also asked similar questions concerning antiepileptic drugs.

Medical students could on average give only 1.8 arguments for, but 2.3 arguments against psychopharmacological treatment. The answers of the psychology students were similar. In contrast, antiepileptic drugs were rated the other way round, more pro arguments were reported. The arguments regarding the antiepileptics could be formulated in a shorter and more precise way than those endorsing psychotropic drugs. Sedation, improvement of anxiety and depressed mood and the fact that psychotropic drugs sometimes are the last option in the treatment of psychiatric disorders are mentioned in favor of psychotropic medication. Negative arguments toward psychotropic medication included that they could be abused by the medical professional by using these drugs to change the feelings of the patient without looking at his 'real problems' (psychotropic drugs as the doctor's 'alibi'). Beside this, a high toxicity and the possibility of changes in the patients personality were mentioned quite often.

The two other questions intended to provoke the students' emotional involvement. The majority showed scepticism towards psychotropic medication by asking for more information about the reasons for prescribing them and thought of consulting other experts. Alternative forms of treatment, especially psychotherapy, were considered and quite often the prescription of psychotropic drugs was rejected. In contrast, the acceptance of antiepileptics was rather positive.

Changes during Undergraduate Medical Education

The attitudes of three groups of medical students at the University of Mainz towards psychotropic drugs were investigated by means of a questionnaire and compared to the general public in 1990/1991 [11, 12]. In this study, questions concerning effects, side effects and indications of psychotropic drugs were combined with questions on treatment with medical drugs in general. Two items discussed a comparison between psychopharmacological and psychotherapeutic treatment and the possibility of a general prohibition of psychotropic medication. The same questions – in the context of an interview – were

Table 1. Medical drugs as seen by different groups of medical students and the general public[1]

	General public	Semester 2–3	7–8	9–10	χ^2 p (2–3 vs. 9–10 semester)
(A) Diseases should be treated with natural remedies and not with chemical drugs	2.4*	2.7	3.6	3.7	0.000
(D) Drugs should only be used in very serious cases	2.2*	2.5	3.1	3.2	0.004
(E) Risks of chemical drugs are as yet underestimated	2.1*	2.1	2.8	2.9	0.001
(F) Taking drugs is an expression of the patient's lack of willpower	3.7*	4.4	4.6	4.6	0.766
(G) Because of modern drugs diseases must no longer be feared	3.7*	4.4	4.7	4.6	0.308

[1] Determined according to a five-point scale from 'I totally agree' (1) to 'I totally disagree' (5).
* $p < 0.001$ vs. students in the 9th to 10th semester.

used in a representative survey of the general public [16]. Three groups of students at different levels of medical education were investigated: (1) students during the preclinical semesters (2nd to 3rd semester; n = 76), (2) students after finishing the first part of the clinical training (7th to 8th semester; n = 128) and (3) students at the end of their clinical training, after finishing the course in psychiatry (9th to 10th semester; n = 119). The clinical training of psychiatry includes 6 courses. A group of 6 students has to interview psychiatric patients. A discussion takes place with an expert regarding psychopathological and therapeutic aspects. The students' attitudes were compared to a subgroup of the public, which had been matched to the students regarding age and education (at least high-school examination; n = 141 [see 11]).

Items showing significant differences between the attitudes of different groups of students and/or the public towards medical treatment are presented in table 1. The public as well as the majority of preclinical medical students prefer a treatment with natural remedies. During medical education, especially in the first clinical semesters in which the course in general pharmacology is offered, attitudes towards medical treatment change significantly: natural remedies are viewed more critically (A). Students become less fearful towards side effects (E) and disagree with the item that medications should only be taken in very serious cases (D). Another group of items, generally supposed

Table 2. Psychopharmacological treatment as rated by different groups of medical students and the public[1]

	Public	Semester 2–3	7–8	9–10	χ^2 p (2–3 vs. 9–10 semester)
Drug treatment is the best way of treating mental illness	3.7	4.1	4.0	3.4	0.001
Drug treatment is the most reliable way of preventing relapse	3.5	3.8	3.8	3.3	0.048
Drug treatment is the treatment most likely to bring about rapid improvement	3.5	3.8	3.8	3.7	0.834
In severe mental illness, drug treatment is the only proper treatment	3.2	4.1	3.9	3.6	0.015
The benefit brought about by drug treatment far outweighs the risk associated with it	3.5	3.5	3.1	2.66	0.001
The cause of mental illness cannot be treated with drugs	2.1	1.6	1.9	2.0	0.126
Drug treatment can only calm patients down	2.3	3.1	4.1	4.4	0.000
Taking drugs helps one to see everything rosier, leaving basic problems unchanged	2.1	2.2	3.0	3.5	0.000
Psychotropic drugs carry a high risk of dependency	1.8	1.5	2.0	2.6	0.000
If taken for long, these drugs can cause irreversible brain damage	2.6	3.0	4.5	3.8	0.001
In the end psychotropic drugs make one even more ill than one was before	2.6	2.9	3.8	4.3	0.000

[1] Determined according to a five-point scale from 'I totally agree' (1) to 'I totally disagree' (5).

to be true by the public, are rejected by all students and do not change during the course of medical education: they do not think that taking medication is a sign of lack of willpower (F) and they do not think either that modern drugs mean a less serious risk of diseases (G).

Table 2 lists the questions on effects and side effects of psychotropic drugs regarding the assumption that modern drugs mean a less serious risk of diseases. Items on therapeutic effectiveness are rated similarly by advanced students and the public, only the preclinical students tend to be more critical. During medical education side effects of psychotropic drugs are increasingly estimated to be a less important problem, according to a more favorable cost/effectiveness calculation. Not only the theoretical courses but also the clinical

Table 3. Effects of courses in psychiatry on attitudes towards a possible prohibition of psychotropic drugs compared with the attitudes of the public (%)

	Public	Semester		
		2–3	7–8	9–10
Generally I prefer a prohibition of these drugs	12.3	2.6	0.8	–
If these drugs cause serious side effects in the long-term outcome, even when they help at the beginning, they should be prohibited	51.1	72.4	59.4	37.8
Generally I am against a prohibition of these drugs	9.4	9.2	18.0	36.1
I'm indecisive	27.2	15.8	21.9	26.1
n (=100%)	141	76	128	119

Answers to the question: Recently a prohibition of psychotropic drugs, used in the treatment of severe psychiatric disorders, was discussed. What do you think about it? Mantel-Haenzel test for linear association: χ^2 MH (1)=6.72, p=0.001.

training contribute to this changing of attitudes. Parallel to this, students realize that psychotropic medication can be used not only to calm patients down, but to treat their symptomatology.

In addition, other aspects of psychopharmacology were investigated [11, 12]: a similarity of these drugs and straitjackets was rejected by the students, but not by the public. That psychiatric patients showing deviant behavior generally should be sedated with psychotropic drugs was more strictly rejected by the students than by the public. All groups did agree with criticism of medical doctors who prefer prescribing psychotropic medication to talking to the patient.

Regarding the question of whether psychotropic drugs should generally be prohibited by law, a significant tendency towards more positive attitudes could be observed during medical education (table 3). Only less advanced students were certain that psychotherapy was generally a better form of treatment than psychopharmacotherapy. Increasingly a more differentiated view on the individual patient developed (table 4).

Discussion

The conclusions of the two studies are quite different: Linden and Becker [10] found that the 'results show that psychopharmaca are mainly criticized', and 'that judgements are based on misinformation and are presented with

Table 4. Effects of courses in psychiatry on students' attitudes towards the treatment with psychotropic drugs versus psychotherapy compared with the attitudes of the public (%)

	General public	Semester		
		2–3	7–8	9–10
Psychotherapy is the better treatment	48.2	33.3	13.4	0.9
Psychopharmacological treatment is the best treatment	4.0	–	–	–
It depends on the type of the psychiatric disorder	21.0	62.3	78.0	88.0
Both treatments are equally good	4.8	2.9	5.5	8.5
I can't decide	22.0	15.8	21.9	26.1
n (=100%)	141	76	128	119

Answers to the question: There can be different opinions about the optimal treatment of psychiatric illnesses. With which of the following opinions do you agree? (students, 2nd to 3rd vs. 9th. to 10th semester: p=0.000, public vs. students 9th to 10th semester: Mantel-Haenzel test for linear association: χ^2 MH(1)=19.67, p=0.000).

much emotional commitment'. Angermeyer et al. [11] and Hillert et al. [12] focus on student scepticism towards psychopharmacology without the interpretation of a general rejection. At least during the course of medical education significant changes towards a more differentiated and positive view were assured.

These differences could be primarily explained by the 7 years between the two investigations as well as by differences between the two universities. The University of Mainz [12] is known to be a center of biological psychiatry, which could explain more favorable attitudes towards psychopharmacology by the students educated at this institution. To avoid premature conclusions, the methodological limitations of psychiatric attitude research have to be considered. The relation between the answers given in questionnaires and the behavior shown in clinical practice remains obscure. Because of the problems arising from the term 'attitudes', especially with professionals and advanced students, it is difficult to define a threshold between knowledge and attitudes.

Attitudes as defined in attitude research, and with this the questions intending to size them up, are of a more general character. In contrast, psychiatric treatment needs to look at the patient's individual aspects. From a clinical and scientific point of view the majority of questions used in attitude questionnaires cannot be answered correctly: any concrete answer would be a wrong one, any question concerning psychotropic drugs would have to be specific because of the very different drugs included in this classification (i.e. benzodiazepines, tricylics, neuroleptics). In the course of their education, medical students are increasingly aware of this aspect. In medical examinations students are trained to read questions in detail. During the course of their medical education the students' situation changes: because of their limited knowledge preclinical students are more able to think that an item like 'psychotropic drugs carry a high risk of dependency' can be rated either with yes or no. After further education students realize that the questionnaire focuses not on knowledge but on something like 'attitudes'. Without discussing every conceivable aspect, there can be no doubt that in any attitude inquiry among experts (like advanced students) there is a thin line between the right answer and a display of abstract bias. The framework of the interviews carried out during a psychiatric education program at the university gives some notion as to the goals of the study.

The other way round, a one-dimensional interpretation of data on whether students approve or disapprove of psychopharmacological treatment may reflect the investigator's subjective point of view and can hardly be objective. To illustrate this problem, investigators should answer their own attitude questions before making the decision of how to interpret the results of the inquiry. Only careful conclusions are justified.

Looking at the differences between the 'attitudes' of the three groups of medical students, the interpretation could not be limited to the simple question of whether 'attitudes' towards psychopharmacological treatment have improved during medical education. The changes in students' points of view have to be considered as well. In this context it has to be pointed out that especially in preclinical students – as well as in the general public – a critical attitude towards psychotropic drugs sometimes can be interpreted as a positive attitude towards psychiatric patients (i.e. the consulting psychiatrist does not abuse their prescription as an 'alibi'). A recent investigation showing that medical students had negative attitudes towards psychiatric patients [17] neglected the methodological limitations of attitude research [18]. During the course of medical education the point of view changes. Growing medical knowledge leads to a more differentiated consideration of pharmacology and psychiatry and with this the problematic aspects of attitude questions.

The 'improvement' of attitudes towards psychopharmacological treatment needs to be seen as the result of a highly complex interaction between the personal situation of the respondent, his medical knowledge and ideological aspects. These parameters, determining the individual's point of view, can also be distinguished in other groups investigated on this subject. The attitudes of psychiatric patients towards psychotropic drugs reflect not only their knowledge about psychotropic medication, but their being inside the disorder and the responsibility taken for their health. Programs to improve the attitudes of patients towards psychiatric treatment therefore need to consider these aspects, if the goal is not just to change answering behavior in attitude questionnaires.

Conclusions

The improvement of the students' attitudes towards psychopharmaco-logical treatment during the course of medical education, especially their rating of side effects as being less striking and a more differentiated view of the individual patient, does not reflect a theoretical but an increasingly practical problem: the responsibilities of a medical doctor. In addition, the majority of the students show a distinct scepticism towards these drugs. Whether or not this is appropriate can only be answered from the individual point of view of the investigator. Only a small group of students reject psychopharmacological treatment by clearly contradicting medical research. The students holding antipsychiatric ideologies, in our study far less than 10%, remain a real problem because of the less rational perception of information and therefore creating a risk of treating their patients inadequately. In further studies it will be useful to focus on this group, looking for their individual characteristics, motives and ideological background. Nevertheless, up to now the very small number, size and strictly German origin of studies on the students' attitudes towards psychopharmacological treatment place considerable limitations on the in-formation acquired.

References

1   Yager J, Lamotte K, Nielsen A, Eaton J: Medical students' evaluation of psychiatry: A cross-country comparison. Am J Psychiatry 1982;139:1003–1009.
2   Gharidian AM, Englesmann F: Medical students' attitude towards psychiatry: A ten-year compar-ison. Med Educ 1982;16:39–43.
3   Wilkinson DG, Greer S, Toone BK: Medical students' attitudes to psychiatry. Psychol Med 1983; 13:185–192.
4   Singer P, Dornbush RL, Brownstein J, Freedman AM: Undergraduate psychiatric education and attitudes of medical students towards psychiatry. Compr Psychiatry 1986;27:14–20.
5   Soufi HE, Raoof AM: Attitude of medical students towards psychiatry. Med Educ 1992;26:38–41.
6   Eagle PE, Marcos LR: Factors in medical students' choice of psychiatry. Am J Psychiatry 1980; 137:423–427.
7   Zimny GH, Sata LS: Influence of factors before and during medical school on choice of psychiatry as a speciality. Am J Psychiatry 1986;143:77–80.
8   Loew TH, Rieger C, Joraschky P, Ebert D, Lungershausen E: Assessment of parts of the medical education by students with and without experience in voluntary history-taking groups: An empirical study. Nervenarzt 1995;66:845–850.
9   Schüppel R, Gatter J, Hrabal V: Teaching psychosomatic medicine: Predictors of students' attitudes towards a compulsory course. J Psychosom Res 1997;42:481–484.
10 Linden M, Becker S: Attitudes and assumptions of medical and psychology students in regard to psychotropic medication. Fortschr Neurol Psychiatr 1984;52:362–369.
11 Angermeyer MC, Matschinger H, Sandmann J, Hillert A: Attitudes of medical students towards the treatment with psychotropic drugs. Comparison between medical students and the general public. Psychiatr Prax 1994;21:58–63.

12 Hillert A, Sandmann J, Angermeyer MC, Däumer R: Medical students' attitude towards psychophar-macotherapy. Changes during the course of medical education. Psychiatr Prax 1994;21:64–69.

13 Kröber HL: Entwarnung quoad '68 und moderne Pharmakotherapie. Einige Meinungen von Medizinstudenten zur Psychiatrie. Spektrum Psychiatr Nervenheilkd 1986;5:187–192.

14 Hillert A, Sandmann J, Ehmig SC, Sobota K, Weisbecker H, Kepplinger HM, Benkert 0: Psychophar-macological drugs as represented in the press. Results of a systematic analysis of newspapers and popular magazines. Pharmacopsychiatry 1996;26:67–71.

15 McPherson IG, Cocks FJ: Attitudes towards mental illness: Influence of data collection procedures. Soc Psychiatry 1983;18:57–60.

16 Angermeyer MC, Däumer R, Matschinger H: Benefits and risks of psychotropic medication in the eyes of the general public; results of a survey in the Federal Republic of Germany. Pharmacopsychia-try 1993;26:114–120.

17 Rössler W, Salize HJ, Trunk V, Voges B: Attitudes of medical students towards the mentally ill. Nervenarzt 1996;67:757–764.

18 Kolodziej ME, Johnson BT: Interpersonal contact and acceptance of persons with psychiatric disorders: A research synthesis. J Consult Clin Psychol 1996;64:1387–1396.

Dr. Dr. Andreas Hillert, Medizinisch-Psychosomatische Klinik Roseneck,
Center for Behavioral Medicine, Am Roseneck 6, D–83209 Prien am Chiemsee (Germany)
Tel. +49 805 1680, Fax +49 805 1683690

Guimón J, Fischer W, Sartorius N (eds): The Image of Madness. The Public Facing Mental Illness and Psychiatric Treatment. Basel, Karger, 1999, pp 197–207

....

Measuring Attitudes toward Psychiatric Medication among Persons with Serious Mental Illness

Jeffrey Draine

School of Social Work, University of Pennsylvania, Philadelphia, Pa., USA

New psychoactive agents have historically been linked to significant changes in the treatment of persons with serious mental illness [1–3]. Most basic texts in psychiatry link the introduction of chlorpromazine to deinstitutionalization. New advances in 'atypical' psychiatric medications for symptoms of schizophrenia are thought to enable community living and stability for those with the most serious illness [4]. While pharmacological research produces new interventions for the biochemical treatment of symptoms, fewer resources are devoted to research for improving the effective delivery of these drugs to consumers [1].

The validity of a medication as a mechanism for clinical change is addressed by efficacy studies, which are tightly controlled randomized clinical trials. In the delivery of the medication to the consumer in the natural service environment, different research questions arise. Medical professionals are often concerned with consumers' compliance with their prescribed medication regimens. Many of the factors that explain compliance are social and psychological in nature, and thus can be very complicated. However, understanding compliance in the natural service environment can potentiate the effectiveness of both medication and psychosocial interventions [3].

Effectiveness studies examine the role of clinical treatment in a social environment. Some may naively understand effectiveness studies to be less rigorous versions of efficacy studies [5]. They are not. Effectiveness studies respond to research questions which differ from efficacy, and which are, by nature, less amenable to conventional methods of rigorous research control. Thus, effectiveness studies may account for complexities in the number of factors, their interaction with one another, and the passage of time in a natural environment. The demand for rigor in the classical sense of the experiment in efficacy studies is replaced by a more elusive demand for conceptual rigor in effectiveness studies.

Compliance can be understood as having at least two components, consumption of the drug, and adherence to a plan of consumption. Consumption of the medication is clearly a factor in effectiveness. Predictable adherence to a plan allows for consumption to be evaluated in an informed way. This need for observation is perhaps at the core of the medical profession's emphasis on compliance in treatment. Some advocates express concern that an undue emphasis on compliance can be coercive. However, if compliance is conceptualized in the context of a professional relationship, then communication between the consumer and the professional is assumed. Thus the plan that is one of the core elements of compliance may be a product of collaboration between clinician and client [6].

Most consumers bring to this collaboration attitudes toward psychiatric medication which are developed through previous treatment experiences. Consumer attitudes are the personal beliefs of consumers about medication. Whether or not consumers believe their medication will control symptoms, decrease the chances of inpatient hospitalization, or improve their lives has an obvious conceptual link to compliance behavior. This link, however obvious, is also complicated. Beliefs or fears about side effects or addiction may also be important. Clinical efforts to increase positive attitudes toward psychiatric medication could improve compliance with medication regimens. Those factors that may plausibly impact consumption, planning, adherence, and attitudes become legitimate targets for interventions to improve the effectiveness of psychiatric treatment with medication.

Linking attitude toward psychiatric medication with compliance behavior can be conceptually challenging. The natural tendency is to predict compliance with positive attitudes. But the temporal order may go in the other direction. Positive attitudes may result from compliant behavior with an efficacious medication. The compliance and the attitude may both be explained by a number of factors associated with health beliefs, such as previous experience, self-efficacy, and socioeconomic status. Likewise negative attitudes may result from noncompliance with a presumably efficacious medication. The consumer does not comply with the treatment, it consequently does not affect symptoms, and thus the consumer concludes that medication is not effective.

This paper reports the use and psychometric testing of a measure of attitudes toward psychiatric medication in three studies of psychosocial services geared toward persons with serious mental illness in the United States. These data will help to meet two research goals: (1) to document reliability of a consumer interview measure of attitudes toward psychiatric medication and (2) to validate this measure with the following hypotheses: positive attitude toward psychiatric medication is positively associated with self-reported compliance with psychiatric medication, and positive attitude toward psychiatric medication is negatively associated with third-party report of noncompliance with psychiatric medication.

Method

The first goal will be met with a principal component factor analysis of data from two of the studies, confirmed with data from the third. Then a multivariate model to explain medication compliance will be constructed and tested against both self-reported compliance and third-party report of noncompliance. Data from the third study will provide the opportunity to test these models. All three studies were randomized field trials. Data used are from baseline interviews, so no intervention effects are inherent in the present analyses.

Overview of the Studies

The first study was a randomized field trial of an assertive community treatment (ACT) model of care for persons with serious mental illness who were also homeless and leaving the Philadelphia jails. Thus, this sample was composed of a population at very high risk for substance abuse problems, housing instability, and thus, noncompliance with medication. Complete sample descriptions and study design can be found elsewhere [7]. The second study was a randomized field trial of ACT delivered by a team of psychiatric consumers as compared to ACT delivered by a team of nonconsumers. Clients for this study were selected from the rolls of a community mental health agency in a culturally and economically diverse section of Philadelphia. Since these clients had not previously been selected for intensive case management services, they tended to be more stable in the community. Therefore, this sample, while diverse, was more typical of urban community mental health clients with serious mental illness. A more complete discussion of this study is also available elsewhere [8].

The third study was a randomized trial of family education services for family members of persons with serious mental illness. Family members who sought services were randomly assigned to individualized consultation, a group workshop or to a wait list control condition. In addition to research involving the families, family members could volunteer contact information for the ill relative in order for researchers to contact them for interviews. Family members were free to refuse contact information and ill relatives were free to refuse participation in the study. Thus, the family member was the primary participant, and the participation of the ill relative was secondary. Among ill relatives contacted, 144 volunteered to be interviewed at baseline. This study was more focused in suburban areas of Philadelphia. Therefore, this sample included more white participants with higher socioeconomic status [9] than the individuals in the first two studies. In the family education study, data are available both from the consumer and from a family member who can independently report medication compliance behavior. Therefore, this study validates a measure of attitudes toward psychiatric medication against third-party report.

Plan for Analysis

All three studies used a measure of attitudes toward medication compliance developed by Streicker and her colleagues [10]. Validation of this measure has not been previously reported. The original version used in the studies included 10 items with a 'strongly agree', 'agree', 'disagree', 'strongly disagree' response scale. Five items were worded positively, and five negatively.

Principal components factor analysis was used to validate the factor structure of the items. Data from the first two studies (the ACT studies) were used for factor analysis. Items that did not load convincingly or consistently on a factor were eliminated until an acceptable factor solution was derived from these data. Then this factor solution was confirmed by using the same items in a factor analysis with data from the third (family education) study. The items were used to compute a variable for attitudes toward psychiatric medication.

This variable was then used in two statistical models explaining compliance with psychiatric medication. The first model explained compliance by self-report from the consumer. The second model explained noncompliance as reported by a third-party family member interviewed at the same point in time (the family member was the primary participant in the family education study). This second model also included consumer self-report as an explanatory variable along with the attitudes toward psychiatric medication variable.

The general model used to explain compliance or noncompliance included sociodemographic characteristics, diagnosis, substance use indicators, homelessness, and symptomatology. Many of these factors have been associated with compliance or noncompliance with the psychiatric medication regimen [2, 3]. Substance use was assessed using the four questions of the CAGE [11], 'Have you ever felt you ought to cut back on your drinking? Have people annoyed you by criticizing your drinking? Have you ever felt bad or guilty about your drinking? Have you ever had a drink first thing in the morning to steady your nerves or get rid of a hangover?' – applying these same items to drug use as well. Any affirmative answer was treated as sign of a problem with alcohol or drugs. Homelessness was simply whether or not the individual had ever been homeless in his or her life. Symptomatology was measured using the Brief Psychiatric Rating Scale [12, 13]. The version used was that developed by Lukoff and his associates [13] specifically for assessing change in psychiatric rehabilitation settings. Subscales were created for Anxiety and Depression, Anergia, Thought Disturbance, Activitation, and Hostile Suspiciousness [14].

Results

Results of Factor Analysis

The 10 items listed in table 1 were entered into a principal components factor analysis with varimax rotation using data from 305 individuals who completed responses to all items in the first two studies (the ACT studies). This analysis produced a two-factor solution in which some items had ambiguous loadings across the two factors. Furthermore, attempts to repeat the analysis within one of the two studies produced three factors with ambiguous loadings. All analyses, however, showed that 5 of the items consistently loaded on the initial factor. Therefore, a factor analysis was attempted which used only these 5 items, and this produced a satisfactory single factor solution that explained 61.8% of the variance among the items. Table 2 reviews the items included in the analysis and the factor loadings. This same solution was produced when

Table 1. Initial items in the attitudes toward psychiatric medication scale (10)

(1)   Psychiatric medication is harmful to your body
(2)   If your symptoms are no longer present, you should discontinue your psychiatric medication
(3)   You dislike taking your psychiatric medication because you have so many side effects
(4)   Taking psychiatric medication interferes with your daily activities
(5)   Taking psychiatric mediation is a necessary part of your rehabilitation
(6)   Taking your psychiatric medication has made it easier for you to deal with your day-to-day stress
(7)   You fear you will become too dependent on your psychiatric medication
(8)   Taking your psychiatric medication prevents you from going to the hospital
(9)   You think your psychiatric medication helps control your symptoms
(10) Taking your psychiatric medication makes you feel better about yourself

Table 2. Factor loadings for final solution

	Item	Factor loading
(5)	Taking psychiatric medication is a necessary part of your rehabilitation	0.758
(6)	Taking your psychiatric medication has made it easier for you to deal with your day-to-day stress	0.838
(8)	Taking your psychiatric medication prevents you from going to the hospital	0.640
(9)	You think your psychiatric medication helps control your symptoms	0.858
(10)	Taking your psychiatric medication makes you feel better about yourself	0.817

the analysis was performed on either of the first two studies alone. Confirmatory factor analysis was then performed on the family education study. This produced the same substantive solution, explaining 58.1% of the variance in the items. Reversing the scoring of the item responses then adding them results in a variable for attitudes toward psychiatric medication where positive values reflect more positive attitudes. In the family education sample, this variable had a mean of 14.57 with a range from 5 to 20. Skewness and kurtosis estimates both indicated that the variable was normally distributed using a $p < 0.10$ standard for non-normality.

Description of the Family Education Study Sample
As indicated above, the sample of consumers used for the second phase of analysis was a sample of secondary participants in a study of services to

family members of persons with serious mental illness. Family members who consented to participate in the study could provide contact information on their ill relatives. A result of this strategy was that the consumers contacted, while they met diagnostic criteria for serious mental illness, were not necessarily engaged in treatment or services for psychiatric disorder. This reduced the influence of a selection factor for greater compliance behavior.

Ill relatives who were eligible had to meet all the following criteria: had a family member who was a participant in the family education study, had in-person or phone contact with their family member at least once a week, lived within a 50-mile radius of Philadelphia, as did their family member, had a major diagnosis of schizophrenia or major affective disorder, had been diagnosed with the disorder at least 6 months before the study and were at least 18 years of age, as were their family members.

Over half of the ill relatives had a schizophrenia diagnosis by report of their family members (58.0, n = 143). Ill relatives reported an average of five lifetime hospitalizations (SD = 5.26) with a range from 0 to 30. Their average age was 34.7 years (n = 144, SD = 10.8) and almost two thirds (63.2%) were male. The average age at first psychiatric hospitalization was 21.91 years (SD = 9.9). Over one fourth (29.9%) reported being homeless at some point in their lives, and 43.4% reported having been arrested. By self-report in response to a direct question, 7.8% of the ill relatives had both drug and alcohol problems. Using the CAGE generated criteria, 44.4% (n = 144) reported some problem related to alcohol and 39.6% (n = 144) reported some problem related to drug use. Exactly half (72 out of 144) of the sample lived with the family member who was the primary participant in the family education study.

Results of Analyses of Hypotheses

The first analysis regressed explanatory variables on the consumers' self-reports of compliance with psychiatric medication regimens. Consumers were asked: 'To what extent do you take your psychiatric medication as prescribed, is it all of the time, most of the time, occasionally, or never?' Among the consumers, 70.8% (n = 102) reported that they took their psychiatric medication as prescribed 'all of the time'. Thus the dependent variable was whether or not the consumer reported compliance all of the time. Table 3 summarizes the results of this analysis. The third row from bottom reviews the change in the −2 log likelihood, an indicator of model fit in logit analysis [15]. Reduction in the −2LL as new blocks of variables are entered can be treated as a statistic which is compared to a χ^2 distribution having degrees of freedom equivalent to the number of variables in the block. Only the last block (1 variable for attitudes toward psychiatric medication) made a statistically significant contribution in the first model. The overall analysis was not statistically significant,

Table 3. Review of logit analysis of self-reported compliance with psychiatric medication (odds ratios; n = 121)

Variable	Step 1	Step 2	Step 3	Step 4	Step 5
Male	0.98	0.94	0.95	0.88	0.87
Age	1.03	1.03	1.03	1.02	1.01
African-American	0.64	0.60	0.56	0.40	0.37
Lives with focus family member	0.68	0.71	0.72	0.73	0.82
Schizophrenia diagnosis		1.28	1.22	1.20	1.19
Ever homeless			0.77	0.87	1.13
Any alcohol problems reported			0.63	0.55	0.54
Any drug problems reported			1.45	1.52	1.59
Anxiety and depression (BPRS)				0.98	0.95
Anergia (BPRS)				1.15	1.22
Thought disorder symptoms (BPRS)				1.05	1.09
Activitation (BPRS)				0.75	0.69*
Hostility (BPRS)				0.90	0.94
Attitudes toward psychiatric medication					1.25**
–2LL as blocks are entered	131.53	131.24	129.86	123.97	115.63
χ^2 for block as entered	4.00	0.29	1.38	5.90	8.34**
χ^2 for model	4.00	4.29	5.67	11.56	19.90

*p < 0.05, **p < 0.01.

χ^2 (d.f.: 14) = 19.90. However, the attitudes toward psychiatric medication variable were statistically significant while controlling for all other explanatory variables. It had an odds ratio of 1.25, indicating that for each increase of 1 in the measure, a consumer was 25% more likely to report full compliance with psychiatric medication. Odds ratios have a value of 1.0 if there is no relationship between variables. Values above 1 indicate the multiple odds that the dependent variable will occur given a 1 point increase in the explanatory variable. Values between 0 and 1 indicate the proportional odds of the negative relationship. Odds ratios above 1.0 are often easier to interpret. The inverse of odds ratios less than 1 (1/x) can be used to transform the statistic to the other direction for easier interpretation, in which case the analyst has to be careful to also conceptually transform the direction of the interpretation.

Table 4 reports the model for noncompliance as reported by the family member. During baseline interviews with family members, they were asked about a list of problems they may have had in the previous month with their ill relative. Among these items was 'noncompliance with prescribed medication'. Thus, the dependent variable for this analysis was family-reported noncompli-

Table 4. Review of logit analysis of family-reported problem with noncompliance (odds ratios; n = 121)

Variable	Step 1	Step 2	Step 3	Step 4	Step 5
Male	0.88	0.77	0.62	0.57	0.58
Age	1.02	1.03	1.03	1.03	1.05*
African-American	1.69	1.45	1.88	2.65	2.46
Lives with focus family member	0.93	1.06	1.01	1.28	1.22
Schizophrenia diagnosis		2.11	2.07	1.78	1.95
Ever homeless			2.38	2.63	2.52
Any alcohol problems reported			1.14	1.05	0.76
Any drug problems reported			1.23	1.81	2.84
Anxiety and depression (BPRS)				1.07	1.08
Anergia (BPRS)				1.12	1.18
Thought disorder symptoms (BPRS)				1.10	1.10
Activitation (BPRS)				0.89	0.82
Hostility (BPRS)				1.23	1.26
Self-reported compliance with psychiatric medication 'all the time'					0.14**
Attitudes toward psychiatric medication					0.79**
−2LL as blocks are entered	142.59	139.70	135.15	122.23	99.19
χ^2 for block as entered	2.96	2.89	4.56	12.91*	23.04***
χ^2 for model	2.96	5.86	10.41	23.33*	46.37***

*p < 0.05; **p < 0.01; ***p < 0.001.

ance. Table 4 reviews the odds ratios for variables in the final model as well as change statistics as block of variables were entered in the model. Only the final two blocks make statistically significant contributions to explaining medication noncompliance. These blocks were one for current symptomatology, and another for attitudes toward psychiatric medication and self-reported compliance. Even when controlling for demographic characteristics, current symptomatology, and self-reported compliance, the measure for attitudes toward psychiatric medication was statistically significant in explaining noncompliance as reported by a family member. The inverse of the odds ratio 0.79 (1/0.79 = 1.26) indicates that for each increase of 1 in the attitude measure, a consumer is 26% more likely to be compliant with prescribed medication by family report of noncompliance. This result controls for a very strong effect for consumer self-report of compliance in the same analysis. The inverse of the odds ratio for consumer self-report of compliance 'all the time' (1/0.14 = 7.14) indicates that when consumers claim complete compliance, they are 7 times more likely to be compliant with prescribed medication by family report of noncompliance.

Discussion

The foregoing analysis demonstrated that consumer attitudes toward psychiatric medication can be reliably and validly measured. Some would expect that the effect for an attitude toward medication measure would actually be measuring the impact of other affective or behavioral concepts, such as self-reported compliance or negative symptoms, toward compliance. However, in this analysis, the attitude measure did accurately explain noncompliance with medication as reported by family members even when controlling for symptoms and consumers' perceptions of their own compliance. The size of the odds ratios associated with attitudes toward medication compliance is particularly noteworthy when considering that they are associated with increases of 1 in a variable normally distributed over a 15-point range (from 5 to 20).

Future studies using this measure could assess more rigorous reliability dimensions. The only dimension assessed here is internal consistency. Attitudes are particularly difficult to measure reliably. Test-retest reliabilities are particularly needed with this interview measure. While interrater reliability is not as important, as this measure requires no rating by an interviewer, they may be effects for interviewer characteristics. There is also a potential social desirability element. Future studies could examine the extent to which socialization into a patient role correlates with reporting more positive attitudes toward psychiatric medication. In the second analysis, this may have been partially addressed by controlling for self-reported compliance 'all the time'.

More substantively, future studies are needed to develop some greater sophistication in modeling compliance behavior among persons with serious and persistent mental illness. Several areas of social science theory, such as health beliefs and coping and adaptation, have sufficient empirical support to guide such a process. The effective delivery of psychiatric drugs is central to the effective delivery of many psychosocial interventions [3]. Thus, research that seeks to understand how these medications are more effectively utilized could potentially improve the quality of life for persons with mental illness [16].

Implied with this optimistic view is an improvement in quality of care. In assessing the impact of attitudes toward medication in explaining the effectiveness of community services, research could assess the interaction of service delivery patterns and qualities with attitudes and outcome. In this process, the value of a process of collaboration with consumers to develop individual medication regimens and enhance consumers' engagement in the clinical process may also be supported [6, 16]. This and other qualities of psychiatric care in the community may develop sufficient support to warrant concrete inclusion in professional practice standards. This would be a step beyond current practice, where collaboration with consumers is lauded as a worthy goal, but its operationalization is rare enough that those clinicians who succeed at it are still perceived by their colleagues as exceptional.

Conclusion

This paper reports the use and psychometric testing of a measure of attitudes toward psychiatric medication in three studies of psychosocial services geared toward persons with serious mental illness in the United States. The analysis demonstrated that consumer attitudes toward psychiatric medication can be reliably and validly measured. The attitude measure did accurately explain noncompliance with medication as reported by family members even when controlling for symptoms and consumers' perceptions of their own compliance. The two main hypotheses were thus confirmed: positive attitude toward psychiatric medication is positively associated with self-reported compliance with psychiatric medication, and negatively associated with third-party report of noncompliance. Future studies are needed to develop some greater sophistication in modeling compliance behavior among persons with serious mental illness.

References

1   Dixon LB, Lehman AF, Levine J: Conventional antipsychotic medications for schizophrenia. Schizophr Bull 1995;21:567–578.
2   Chen A: Noncompliance in community psychiatry: A review of clinical interventions. Hosp Community Psychiatry 1991;42:282–287.
3   Draine J, Solomon P: Explaining attitudes toward medication compliance among a seriously mentally ill population. J Nerv Ment Dis 1994;182:50–54.
4   Buchanan RW: Clozapine: Efficacy and safety. Schizophr Bull 1995;21:579–592.
5   Hogarty GE, Schooler NR, Baker RW: Efficacy versus effectiveness. Psychiatr Serv 1997;48:1107.
6   Draine J, Solomon P: Coercion of consumers to comply with treatment in community care: Collaboration among consumers, families, and professionals. Continuum 1997;4:39–50.
7   Solomon P, Draine J: One year outcomes of a randomized trial of case management with seriously mentally ill clients leaving jail. Eval Rev 1995;19:256–273.
8   Solomon P, Draine J: The efficacy of a consumer case management team: Two year outcomes of a randomized trial. J Ment Health Adm 1995;22:135–146.
9   Solomon P, Draine J, Mannion E, Meisel M: Effectiveness of two models of brief family education: Retaining gains by family members of adults with serious mental illness. Am J Orthopsychiatry 1997;67:221–234.

10   Streicker SK, Amdur M, Dincin J: Educating patients about psychiatric medications: Failure to enhance compliance. Psychosoc Rehabil J 1986;9:15–28.
11   Mayfield D, McCleod G, Hall P: The CAGE questionnaire: Validation of a new alcoholism screening questionnaire. Am J Psychiatry 1974;131:1121–1123.
12   Overall J, Gorhom D: The Brief Psychiatric Rating Scale. Psychol Rep 1962;10:799–812.
13   Lukoff D, Lieberman RP, Nuechterlein DK: Symptom monitoring in the rehabilitation of schizophrenia patients. Schizophr Bull 1986;12:578–602.
14   Guy W: ECDEU Assessment Manual for Psychopharmacology. Rockville, National Institute for Mental Health, 1976.
15   Agresti A: Categorical Data Analysis. New York, Wiley, 1990.
16   Diamond R: Drugs and the quality of life: The patients' point of view. J Clin Psychiatry 1985;46: 145–159.

Prof. Jeffrey Draine, Assistant Professor, School of Social Work, University of Pennsylvania, 3701 Locust Walk, Philadelphia, PA 19104 (USA)
Tel. +1 610 573 9298, Fax +1 610 573 2099

Guimón J, Fischer W, Sartorius N (eds): The Image of Madness. The Public Facing Mental Illness and Psychiatric Treatment. Basel, Karger, 1999, pp 208–215

Psychoeducational Groups in Schizophrenic Patients

Iñaki Eguiluz [a, b], *Miguel Angel González Torres* [a, b], *José Guimón* [b]

[a] Department of Neuroscience, Section of Psychiatry,
  University of the Basque Country and
[b] Psychiatry Service, Basurto Hospital, Bilbao, Spain
[c] Department of Psychiatry, University of Geneva, Switzerland

Since 1896, when Kraepelin identified the schizophrenic disorder, until today, part of the stigma which has been traditionally associated with the disorder based on its supposed incurability. This pessimistic outlook is not only perceptible among the laypeople, but even among nonspecialist doctors and among psychiatrists who continue to rigidly believe that if a schizophrenic person is cured, it was not really 'authentic schizophrenia' and the diagnosis should be reviewed.

At present, the efficiency of neuroleptic medication in the treatment of schizophrenia is unquestionable, as shown by several studies [1, 2]. Consequently, over the past few decades hopes have been raised for changes in both the prognosis of the illness and the quality of life of patients, and admissions into psychiatric institutions have fallen significantly, as reflected in the so called deinstitutionalization process [3].

Nevertheless, every day we are still faced with extremely worrying facts: 50% of all schizophrenic patients suffer relapses in the first year following their last episode [4]. These patients spend between 15 and 20% of their time in institutions as a result of the frequent occurrence of relapses [5, 6].

There are numerous factors which influence the development of these relapses, although it is not the aim of this paper to carry out such an analysis. One of the main reasons for the high rate of relapses in conventional treatment, is the patients' failure to comply with the medication. Only 40–50% of patients properly follow the therapeutic indications related to medication [7], this failure rate reaching up to 75% in patients who are suffering a first episode [4].

Furthermore, this fact is not a phenomenon unique to schizophrenic patients. In a prior study carried out in our area [8], we observed that the attitude of the general population towards psychoactive drugs was negative. This situation directly influences psychiatric treatment and schizophrenia in particular, where genetic components (relatives with a similar diagnosis), and an insufficient awareness of the illness on the part of the vast majority of patients lead to a poor medication compliance [9].

During the last few years several studies have been aimed at improving the treatment compliance of schizophrenic patients [10–18]. All of them conclude that setting up psychoeducational groups for schizophrenic patients and their relatives leads to better medication compliance and, secondly, a significant reduction in the number of relapses and hospital readmissions.

Psychoeducational groups have been run in the Basurto Hospital in Bilbao for schizophrenic patients and their relatives since 1991. The experience is at the same time also used as an alternative to classic outpatient treatment. The opinion is unanimous that psychoeducational groups are more effective when relatives as well as patients participate. There is doubt as to whether it is better for them to form joint or separate groups. Joint groups can become family therapy groups which is not our objective.

Materials and Methods

All the patients who took part in the study came from the Inpatient Psychiatric Unit at the Basurto General Hospital. The only criterion for inclusion was 'difficulty' in complying with medication, which had been assessed both in the inpatient unit and from medical records from their mental health center.

Given the great degree of heterogeneity among the patients, two groups were established: group 1: patients with a diagnosis of a schizophreniform disorder or schizophrenic disorder with less than 1 year evolution according to DSM-III-R criteria; all of them were first-episode psychotic patients, and group 2: patients with a diagnosis of schizophrenic disorder with more than 1 year evolution according to DSM-III-R criteria. For reasons mentioned above, additional two groups were set up separately for patients' relatives. The groups were open and their number varied between 8 and 10 patients per group. They met every fortnight, with the session lasting an hour for each group. The family groups met every 2–3 months.

Creation of structure was carried out according to Yalom's model [19]. Although this structure was feasible in the first few weeks, subsequently, while maintaining the same philosophy, the meetings became less structured and 'freer'. The groups were run by a psychiatrist from the Psychiatry Service with a 4th year intern (resident) participating on a rota basis.

An agreement was drawn up for group 1, which varied between 1.5 and 2 years, following the guidelines set in the Bruges Consensus Conference, for the patients with first psychotic episodes. When this period was over, if the evolution had been satisfactory, the medication was progressively removed (3–5 months), and the patients were referred to the outpatient unit. In the case of group 2, given the chronic nature of their pathology, patients were invited to participate in the project indefinitely, with the option of leaving whenever they thought best.

BPRS, PANSS, CGI and Simpson-Angus scales were used to assess the patients. The administration of these scales was carried out on joining the project, every 6 months and whenever these was a relapse. The BPRS scale [20] was used as relapse criteria. The three BPRS-positive psychotic items (hallucinations, thought content and disorganized thought) were assessed independently; a score of 6–7 for any of the three symptoms meant a relapse. As the inpatient unit was the starting point for all the participants, at the time the project got under way, the BPRS total scores were equal to or more than 30 and the CGI score did not exceed the 'averagely ill' classification.

A group of 40 patients with the same diagnosis who had been discharged from our unit in 1990 were chosen retrospectively as a control sample, before starting the follow-up psychoeducational groups. Data was collected on the patients who had an adequate diagnosis going back in time, from the starting date of the groups until 40 were selected, a similar number of patients as that in the psychoeducational groups. The analysis involved registering data on the sex and age of each patient, and in addition it was established whether it was his or her first episode by consulting the clinical records. Subsequently, available databases were consulted to find out how many readmissions each patient had registered from 1991 until commencement of the study.

The comparative analysis was carried out using the following variables: sex, age, whether or not it was the first episode which had been the reason for their inclusion in the study and the number of readmissions between 1991 and September 1996. This last variable is the result or main outcome. We followed a nonrandomized open clinical trial methodology, which can be regarded as a pilot study prior to the wider and more rigorous research, that is now in the first phases of development.

The t test was used for the statistical analysis in order to compare averages in independent samples with a normal variable distribution, χ^2 to compare proportions and the Mann-Whitney U test to make comparisons of averages in independent samples for cases where a normal distribution of the variable could not be assumed. In the analysis which employed the t test, the calculation of the confidence interval at 95% was also carried out.

Results

If we analyze the group and control samples (standard treatment) together, we obtain the data which appear in table 1 for the main variables. We must point out the significant differences in age (the patients in the psychoeducational groups were younger than the control group patients) and the number of readmissions registered in the study period (patients treated in psychoeducational groups were readmitted less often than patients in the control group). It is interesting to note that the distribution by sex and the proportion of first episodes do not show significant differences between the two groups.

The data in the two groups of patients have been separated according to whether they are first episode cases or not and appear in table 1 (first episodes) and table 1 (record of previous episodes). By selecting the first episodes of

Table 1. Age, sex and mean number of admissions according to the type of group

	n	Age	Sex (% male)	1st episode (%)	Admissions 1991–1996
General					
Psychoeducational group	39	27.8 (4.30)	61.5	53.8	0.30 (1.17)
Control group	40	35.77 (9.32)[a]	65.0 (NS)	47.4 (NS)	2.32 (1.92)[b]
First episodes					
Psychoeducational group	21	24.9 (2.40)	52.4		0.04 (0.21)
Control group	18	34.22 (7.61)[a]	61.1 (NS)		1.61 (1.24)[b]
Patients with previous episodes					
Psychoeducational group	18	31.27 (3.39)	72.2		0.61 (1.68)
Control group	20	37.75 (10.67)[a]	65.0 (NS)		3.05 (2.25)[b]

Age and admission values represent means with SD in parentheses. NS = Not significant.
[a] t test; p < 0.001.
[b] U Mann-Whitney; p < 0.0001.

both samples we find a similar proportion according to sex and a higher age for patients in the control sample with standard treatment. In addition, a very significant difference is to be noted in the number of readmissions for the period 1991–1996, with the average number of readmissions 40 times greater for patients in the control sample in relation to those in the psychoeducational group. By selecting the patients who have suffered from previous episodes we can observe a similar proportion of men and women and a higher age for the control sample undergoing standard treatment. The difference in terms of readmissions is important (5 times greater for the control group) and very significant from a statistical point of view.

In order to analyze the influence of the sex variable, an assumption considered to be important, we compared the number of admissions for men and women without considering the type of treatment and the previous evolution (table 2). Then we compared men and women separately for first episode cases and for those having had previous episodes.

We can observe that the development of the number of readmissions for men and women is similar; no statistically significant differences are to be found either by studying all the patients together without taking their previous medical record into account or by separating them according to whether or not they suffered previous episodes. It also seems relevant to point out that the age of men and women is similar for the three groups.

Table 2. Age and mean number of admissions by sex

	n	Age	Admissions 1991–1996
General			
Men	50	31.76 (6.95)	1.32 (1.65)
Women	29	32.03 (10.28) (NS)	1.34 (2.25) (NS)
First episodes			
Men	23	30.27 (8.30)	0.95 (0.79)
Women	17	27.82 (5.22) (NS)	0.52 (1.36) (NS)
Patients with previous episodes			
Men	27	33.15 (5.54)	1.61 (1.89)
Women	12	38.00 (12.77) (NS)	2.50 (3.08) (NS)

Values represent means with SD in parentheses. NS = Not significant.

Discussion

The fact that the study is a nonrandomized pilot study limits the possibilities of extrapolating the data obtained. Two methodological aspects stand out above the rest in our opinion: the selection of the control sample and age.

Patients who joined the psychoeducational groups were selected expressly according to the criteria described in the Materials and Methods section. This led us to question whether the data could be compared with that pertaining to nonselected patients, so we decided as an alternative to select a sample of patients with the same diagnoses and who had been admitted to our unit before the two groups started. In this way, we had a degree of certainty that at least some of the control patients were similar to those who months later would be selected for the group follow-up. At the time of calculating the number of readmissions, the control group patients were not interviewed, data were instead consulted from the available databases. This obviously means that there is a risk that admissions which were not clearly reflected in the documentation may have been missed and that the number of readmissions in the control group could possibly be higher. Rather than weakening our conclusions, however, this on the contrary strengthens them, because the differences in the number of readmissions could be even greater.

The age of the psychoeducational group sample patients is different to that of the control sample patients; viewed both globally and as discrete groups according to whether they are first episode patients or not, those subjects attending the groups are younger than control patients. A higher age could be thought to entail more readmissions as from a certain moment. Although this has been highly debated in recent literature, it is true that the age difference is a relevant difference in the study. In studies subsequent to this pilot analysis, we will have to treat age as a possible source of differences and adjust the methodology of the study to solve this problem. The results of the psychoeducational groups' experience with schizophrenic patients seem clear-cut and are confirmed in other similar experiences and mentioned earlier in this paper.

At present, most professionals agree that treatment compliance is one of the main problems to be solved in order to reduce the rate of relapse in schizophrenic patients. In addition, we find ourselves before the development of new molecules for the treatment of schizophrenia, which makes us feel extremely optimistic, although the benefit will be scarce for the patients if they do not comply with the treatment.

There are numerous factors which lead to the noncompliance of these patients: general attitude towards psychoactive drugs, scarce awareness of the illness, fear of adverse effects, lack of information on the illness and lack of support from relatives. A classic approach to the illness, which limits therapy to isolated and individual action by the doctor with the patient, often turns out to be insufficient, to deal with the number of complex and varied situations. Setting up 'psychoeducational groups' may be a suitable means to develop a multidisciplinary program both for patients and their relatives.

We have always defended the idea that the optimum treatment for schizophrenia involves a combination of psychosocial and psychopharmacological interventions. Although it has never been our intention to use the groups for psychotherapy, it cannot be denied that this occurs in some way. We share the opinions of authors such as Gomes-Schwartz [21] and Mueser and Berenbaum [22], who state that psychodynamically oriented psychotherapy is not suitable for schizophrenic patients.

Nevertheless, certain aspects of supportive psychotherapy (strengthening interpersonal relationships, help to manage life tensions, improving social functioning, building up self-esteem) may be present in the groups and clearly influence development, because the basis for support psychotherapy, as in all doctor-patient relationships, is a therapeutic alliance, the cornerstone of medical practice in general and of the treatment of chronic illnesses such as schizophrenia in particular. This relationship, as stated by Herz [23], is a fundamental strategy in the prevention of relapses, as prodromal signs may be detected with greater ease by both patients and their relatives.

Finally, another fundamental aspect in current medical practice is that of cost analysis. There are numerous macroeconomics studies on the cost of schizophrenia. This disorder generates higher direct costs than any other mental disorder, as a result of psychiatric admissions and the community treatment they necessitate. The majority of these costs can be traced to the group of patients with the worst results [24, 25]. Any therapeutical activity directed at the prevention of relapses and, consequently, the reduction of the number of psychiatric admissions will coincide with the modern health management models towards which we are inevitably heading.

References

1   Davis JM: Antipsychotic drugs; in Freedman AM, Sadock BJ (eds): Comprehensive Textbook of Psychiatry. Baltimore, Williams & Wilkins, 1980, vol 3, pp 2257–2289.
2   Kane JM: Treatment of schizophrenia. Schizophr Bull 1987;13:133–156.
3   Dencker SJ, Dencker K: Does community care reduce the need for psychiatric beds for schizophrenic patients? Acta Psychiatr Scand 1994(suppl 382):74–79.
4   Gaebel W, Pritzker A: One year outcome of schizophrenic patient, the interaction of chronicity and neuroleptic treatment. Pharmacopsychiatry 1985;18:235–239.
5   Maurer K, Biehl H: Klinikaufenthalt und produktive Rückfälle bei ersterkrankten Schizophrenen. Determinanten des Zeitverlaufs zwischen stationären Aufnahmen bzw. schizophrenen Reziduven über fünf Jahre. Nervenheilkunde 1988;7:279–290.
6   Gmür M, Tschopp A: Die Behandlungskontinuität bei schizophrenen Patienten in der Ambulanz. Eine Fünfjahresnachuntersuchung. Nervenarzt 1988;59:727–730.
7   Kissling W: Directrices para la prevención de recidivas de la esquizofrenia con neurolépticos. Barcelona, Springer Ibérica, 1994.
8   Guimón J, Ozamiz A, Viar I: Actitudes de la población ante el consumo terapéutico de psicofármacos. VII Reunión de la Sociedad Española de Psiquiatría Biológica. 1980, pp 165–175.
9   Ulmar G, Ullrich J, Starzinski T: Attitudinal change of involuntary schizophrenic patients. Fortschr Neurol Psychiatr 1995;63:480–486.
10 Eguiluz I: Evolución actitudinal y clínica de pacientes esquizofrénicos a través de su participación en grupos de medicación; doctoral dissertation, Universidad del País Vasco, Bilbao, 1987.
11 Schooler NR, Keith SJ: Role of medication in psychosocial treatment, in Herz MI, Keith SJ, Docherty JP (eds): Psychosocial Treatment of Schizophrenia. Amsterdam, Elsevier, 1990, pp 45–67.
12 Anderson CM, Hogarty GE, Reiss DJ: Psychoeducational family management of schizophrenia; in Herz MI, Keith SJ, Docherty JP (eds): Psychosocial Treatment of Schizophrenia. Amsterdam, Elsevier, 1990, pp 153–166.
13 Guimón J, Eguiluz I, Bulvena A: Group pharmacotherapy in schizophrenics: Attitudinal and clinical changes. Eur J Psychiatry 1993;7:147–154.
14 Bäuml J, Kissling W, Buttner P, Pitschel-Walz G, Welschhold M, Bender W: Informationszentrierte Gruppen für schizophrene Patienten und deren Angehörige – Akzeptanz, Effizienz und Durch-führrbarkeit unter klinischen Routinebedingungen. Schizophrenie 1994:6–14.
15 Kissling W: Compliance, quality assurance and standards for relapse prevention in schizophrenia. Acta Psychiatr Scand 1994(suppl 382):16–24.
16 Kieserg A, Hornoug WP: Psychoedukatives Training für schizophrene Patienten. Ein verhaltensther-apeutisches Behandlungsprogramm zur Rezidivprophylaxe. Tübingen, DGVT, 1994.
17 McGorry PD: Psychoeducation in first-episode psychotic patients: A therapeutic process. Psychiatry 1995;58:313–328.
18 Goldstein MJ: Psychoeducation and relapse prevention. Int Clin Psychopharmacol 1995(suppl 5): 59–69.
19 Yalom ID: Inpatient Group Psychotherapy. New York, Basic Books, 1985.
20 Nuechterlein KH, Davson ME: Developmental processes in schizophrenic disorders. Longitudinal studies of vulnerability and stress. Schizophr Bull 1992;18:387–425.
21 Gomes-Schwartz B: Individual psychotherapy of schizophrenia; in Bellack AS (ed): Schizophrenia: Treatment, Management and Rehabilitation. New York, Grune & Stratton, 1984, pp 307–335.

22   Mueser KT, Berenbaum H: Psychodynamic treatment of schizophrenia. Is there a future? Psychol Med 1990;20:253–262.
23   Herz MI: Early intervention in schizophrenia; in Herz MI, Keith SJ, Docherty JP (eds): Psychosocial Treatment of Schizophrenia. Amsterdam, Elsevier, 1990, pp 25–44.
24   Davies LM, Drummond MF: Assessment of costs and benefits of drug therapy for treatment-resistant schizophrenia in the United Kingdom. Br J Psychiatry 1993;162:38–42.
25   Drummond MF: Cost of illness studies. A major headache? Pharmacoeconomics 1992;2:1–4.

Dr. Iñaki Eguiluz, Fundación OMIE, Manuel Allende 19-1°-bis,
E–48010 Bilbao (Spain)
Tel. +34 94 443 90 49, Fax +34 94 422 38 24

Guimón J, Fischer W, Sartorius N (eds): The Image of Madness. The Public Facing Mental
Illness and Psychiatric Treatment. Basel, Karger, 1999, pp 216–221

························

Neuroleptics: The Point of View of Consumers and Their Families

Anne Spagnoli

GRAAP Patient Relatives Group, Lausanne, Switzerland

The GRAAP (Groupe d'accueil et d'action psychiatrique/a support and
action group for people with psychiatric problems) in Lausanne is an association with about 600 members, all of whom are either users of psychiatric
services or patients' relatives [see 1]. The following remarks are the result of
the experience acquired as the activity coordinator of the GRAAP patient
relatives' group.

The Weight of Experience

Obviously, neuroleptics occupy an important place in the lives of those who
have to take them regularly. This issue is often discussed in our association, and
we frequently invite professionals who can give advice and answer our questions
concerning different kinds of treatment and medication. These discussions are
usually lively and controversial, and they reveal a wide range of opinions and
attitudes. But then, of course, for psychiatric patients the issue of neuroleptics
is neither academic nor theoretical; their ideas about the subject are usually the
result of one or more very concrete and often painful personal experiences.

They have to deal with the practical inconvenience of having to take their
medication regularly and at the right time. More important, they have to put
up with the disagreeable side effects neuroleptics may provoke – and the variety
of these side effects is probably richer than officially documented. And they
have to live with the risk – however remote – of serious and irreversible side
effects such as tardive dyskinesia. One should add that because neuroleptics
are supposed to modify not only our behavior but also our way of perceiving
the world, they can be experienced as being very alienating.

Users of psychiatric services are therefore understandably irritated when professionals make disparaging remarks, underrating the scope and the painfulness of the side effects and unthinkingly repeat smug clichés such as: 'but it is for your own good ...'. I am sure that the psychiatrist from Lausanne who used to try out neuroleptics on himself before prescribing them was not tempted to make this kind of remark!

Neuroleptics Do Have Disagreeable Effects, But ...

So neuroleptics are indeed an important issue for psychiatric patients and their relatives, and, because of their being a daily experience, their negative aspects are often mentioned. But other aspects are also discussed such as how long neuroleptics should be taken and if and when taking them may be interrupted without suffering dire consequences. Our members are also interested in finding out about possible alternative treatments. In the GRAAP's 1996 annual congress, representatives of different types of medicine (homeopathic medicine, massage, traditional Chinese and Ayurvedic medicines) were invited to explain how they could help psychiatric patients. One of the conclusions of this congress was that, although many of these treatments could help patients and improve their comfort, they could not as yet replace neuroleptic medication, but only complement it.

Most members of the GRAAP admit that in spite of their inconveniences and side effects, neuroleptics are useful since they calm down some symptoms and some of the anguish caused by mental illness, thus allowing people suffering from psychosis to communicate more easily and to reach some social integration.

In our association we are well aware that when a patient is undergoing a crisis he will often flatly refuse to take neuroleptics or any other medication for that matter – when he feels anxious and persecuted. However, a skilful therapist should be able to reassure him and persuade him to accept the treatment. And when this patient feels better, he will often admit that the neuroleptics, however disagreeable, can be helpful. However, it must be stressed that the benefits of neuroleptic medication are often more readily perceived by the patient's relatives and caregivers than by the patient himself.

Are We Really Talking about Neuroleptics Here?

Often, while apparently discussing neuroleptics, many other issues are addressed. It seems to be easier to discuss pills, injections, dosages and side effects rather than talking about feelings and emotions. But feelings and emotions tend to creep back and confuse the issues. For example, some patients still get the first inkling of their diagnosis by reading the pharmaceutical prospectus. Here neuroleptics become a devious way of finding out a 'truth' they may feel is being withheld. In other cases, people will try to use the neuroleptics to measure the seriousness of someone's illness: 'He is taking 100 mg, he must be quite mad.' Sometimes neuroleptics are used as a threat: 'If you don't obey, we will have to give you an injection.' When a patient is feeling better, the neuroleptics may become a permanent reminder of an illness he would rather forget about. Doctors and nurses may be tempted to judge a patient's value as a person by his degree of 'compliance' where neuroleptics are concerned. A psychiatrist can give lengthy answers to his patient's questions about neuroleptics, but if he has not heard the underlying question: 'Doctor, how seriously ill am I? Will I get better?', this therapist's explanations will probably be quite inadequate. In these different examples, neuroleptics are obviously not the real issue, but it is doubtful whether everyone concerned will be aware of this.

Of course the above remarks can be made concerning nearly any medication, but where psychiatric illnesses are concerned, the emotional dimension and the quality of the relationship between doctors and patients are particularly important.

Doctor-Patient Relationship

Users of psychiatric services and their relatives are of course interested in the different aspects of neuroleptics, but they are particularly sensitive about what one could call the 'human relations' aspect. When the therapist prescribed the drug, did he give the patient the necessary explanations? Has the patient been able to explain his point of view to the therapist and have his arguments been listened to? Is he sure he can reach his therapist or some other caregiver if he is anxious about the effects of a new medication? What do his relatives think of his medication and how well informed are they?

Users of psychiatric services often have the impression that any reservation patients express concerning neuroleptics is interpreted as a rebellion against medical authority, or even as a symptom of a relapse. The logical consequence of this is that dosages are increased and whatever the patient is trying to say is totally rejected. In our opinion therapists should be able to discuss medication with their patients and accept the latter's unwillingness to take neuroleptics without immediately reacting as though this reluctance was a challenge to their authority.

Especially where medication is concerned, therapists still seem to value 'compliance', which is often nothing more than passive obedience, above a more active if less submissive attitude. But is passive obedience really the attitude which will best help a person overcome the difficulties of a psychiatric illness? The therapist's general attitude, and how he relates to his patient, is also important.

For example, mental health specialists and researchers have all kinds of disagreements over treatments, medication and diagnosis. When these quarrels find their way out of faculties and institutes and are relayed by the media, psychiatric patients will sometimes use such information to argue against the medication chosen by their own therapists. Instead of taking offence, the latter could seize the opportunity to encourage their patients to be more critical and better informed.

What about Patients' Relatives?

Many users of psychiatric services live with their families or keep in touch with them. The burden of caring for a mentally ill patient at home is considerable, but professionals often seem unaware of this and sometimes even add to this burden. For instance, psychiatrists often give relatives the responsibility for seeing that their patients take their medication correctly.

But this can be a very difficult and tricky responsibility for family members.

I remember how distressed I was when I was told to make sure my husband took his neuroleptics: though I was not told what he was suffering from or what would happen if he did not take his pills. I have seen middle-aged parents feel terribly guilty because they had been unable to persuade their grown-up son to take his neuroleptics. Obviously, here again, the real problem has very little to do with neuroleptics, and everything with the relationship that has been achieved between the therapist, the patient and his family.

Relatives tend to be ambivalent toward neuroleptics. On the one hand, these pills and injections make their lives easier by reducing some of the symptoms. In the GRAAP's group of relatives I have heard family members talking of neuroleptics as though they were real life buoys, and they are prepared to go to any lengths and to use every trick to make the sick person take his medication. On the other hand, relatives are well placed to realize how disagreeable the side effects can be: they have seen their child, their spouse or their parent drag around with jerky movements, sleepy and apathetic because of heavy medication, and they can therefore be tempted to encourage the patient to refuse them.

Thus neuroleptics can become an opportunity for relatives to rally the cause of their patient against the medical team, or on the contrary an excuse to support the therapist 'against' the patient. Obviously, this kind of problem cannot be solved simply by giving out information. It must be dealt with in a global approach in which relatives – as well as patients – are considered as partners, and in which their own specific problems and needs are addressed.

Some Examples of What We Feel Should Change

People who are taking neuroleptics of course hope that research will eventually produce medication with fewer – or no – side effects. Or that research in chronobiology, for instance, will gradually allow a decrease in the dosages. But in the meanwhile, patients ask that professionals and researchers take the time to listen to them, to take their experience into account, and to consider them as partners in the difficult struggle against mental illness. And this includes changing the different aspects of doctor-patient relationship as previously suggested.

Learning about Neuroleptics

Psychiatric patients need to know why neuroleptics are prescribed, and what effects an increase or a decrease in the dosages can have, so that they may take an active part in their treatment and become more autonomous. Psychoeducational groups aimed at learning how to deal with the medication already exist in some institutions, but they could be developed further with the possibility of becoming more detached from the institutions.

Medication Is Not Enough

Neuroleptics are useful because they suppress certain symptoms, but this fact seems to encourage caregivers to focus only on what is *wrong* with their patients. No human being can be reduced to his symptoms and handicaps, however serious. Even the sickest person also has resources that can be important in the struggle against his illness – personal resources as well as the resources of his social environment, for instance. That is why we think that the prescription of neuroleptics should always be considered as part of a therapeutic project.

What Kind of Therapeutic Project?

In our opinion a therapeutic project is not just what the doctor decides concerning his patient's treatment. However learned, a therapist cannot decide what is good for 'his' patient, or what he should be like, or where he should go. His job is to help the mentally ill person to discover his own resources and his own limits, to help him see which paths are open to him, and which ones it would be safer to avoid so that the patient can gradually find his own way. In other words, the therapeutic project should be the result of a negotiation between the therapist, the patient and – unless the patient objects – his close relatives. We sometimes call this partnership a 'trialog'.

Self-Help Groups

I would like to conclude in stressing how important it is for patients and their relatives to get together and organize self-help groups. When the users of psychiatric services can discuss their experiences and their problems amongst themselves, they help each other in learning to deal with their illness and their suffering; friendship and solidarity can be precious allies in the struggle against some of the dire consequences of mental illness. Relatives can also learn to cope with the burden of caring for a mentally ill person and be encouraged to reorganize their lives, for example so as to avoid overinvolvement with him.

In these groups, patients and their relatives can also gain more confidence, so as to be able to express their needs and their hopes without feeling intimidated by the medical and scientific establishment. And this can be very positive for all parties involved.

References

1   Pont M: Stigmatization and Destigmatization: The Point of View of Psychiatric Patients and Their Families; in Guimón J, Fischer W, Sartorius N (eds): The Image of Madness. Basel, Karger, 1999, pp 138–142.

Anne Spagnoli, Av. Denantou 23, CH–1006 Lausanne (Switzerland)
Tel./Fax +41 21 616 6377

Guimón J, Fischer W, Sartorius N (eds): The Image of Madness. The Public Facing Mental
Illness and Psychiatric Treatment. Basel, Karger, 1999, pp 222–230

....

The Role of Communication and Physician-Patient Collaboration: Enhancing Adherence with Psychiatric Medication[1]

M. Robin DiMatteo

Department of Psychology, University of California, Riverside, Calif., USA

The past half century has brought tremendous developments in the care
of psychiatric illnesses. New medications provide the opportunity to alleviate
suffering and improve patients' quality of life. The correct use of these medications by patients is not, however, something that can be taken for granted.
Despite the capacity of these medications to control conditions that were once
uncontrollable, many patients ignore their physicians' directives and fail to
take their prescribed medications [1, 2].

The problem of patient noncompliance with medication is not confined
to the realm of psychiatric care. An average of 38% of patients are noncompliant with short-term medication prescriptions and over 43% with longer-term
treatments. These disturbingly high percentages are actually likely to be under-
estimates [3].

Noncompliance involves a patient altering the recommended dosage and
timing of his or her medication, or otherwise using the medication in such a
way as to pose a threat to health [4]. Noncompliant patients come from all
backgrounds and education levels, and most tend to hide adherence problems,
fearing physician reprimand or displeasure [5]. As a result, physicians may be
confused in the diagnostic process, drawing incorrect conclusions based upon

[1] The author wishes to thank the Health and Behavior Research Network of the John
D. and Catherine T. MacArthur Foundation, and the Center for Social and Behavioral
Sciences of the College of Humanities, Arts, and Social Sciences and the Center for Ideas
and Society at the University of California, Riverside Calif. for continuing support of her
research on patient adherence.

patients' 'responses' to drugs not taken and procedures not followed. Noncompliance can also be dangerous for patients when their physicians increase dosages or change medications not knowing that the initial prescriptions were not taken. In general, poor adherence can lead to poor health care outcomes and possibly to severely interrupted lives.

The very act of being adherent, on the other hand, can be beneficial to many patients. Research subjects who are adherent tend to have better outcomes than those who are not, regardless of regimen (real treatment or placebo) [6]. This suggests that adherent patients may have more positive expectations that serve as a self-fulfilling prophecy. Commitment to a treatment regimen may lead to feelings of greater well-being and confidence, and better health habits.

Reasons for Noncompliance

Patients rarely adhere to recommended treatments because of simple deference to their 'doctor's orders'. Instead, they attempt to decide quite rationally what they will and will not do to take care of themselves. Their decisions are typically based upon two kinds of beliefs about the recommended treatment: in its value (whether the benefits outweigh the costs) and in its expected efficacy (the likelihood of attaining the desired outcome) [7]. With or without their physician's participation, most patients weigh the costs (broadly defined in terms of finances, time, inconvenience) of each treatment against the benefits they expect to obtain. Some patients are noncompliant because the personal and social circumstances of their lives make adherence impossible. Patients must sometimes choose to satisfy other demands over the physician's recommendation for a health care action.

Some reasons for noncompliance are less straightforward than disbelief and practical difficulty. Patients may choose not to adhere to their treatment as a way of denying their disease. Their failure to comply may represent a breaking of the symbolic rules of a system that tells them they are dependent and under the control of a powerful authority figure, the physician. Patients may fail to comply in order to retain the ultimate ability to decide for themselves the course of action they believe is in their own best interest.

Physician-Patient Relationship

'All medical care flows through the relationship between physician and patient, and the spoken word is the most important tool in medicine' [8]. This statement may be even more true in psychiatry than in other specialties; the relationship between psychiatrist and patient has traditionally been recognized as central to the delivery of care. As psychiatric care benefits from developing psychoactive pharmacology, and as some managed care protocols reduce time spent with patients, the pressures toward dispensing medications with little development of the therapeutic relationship remains a danger. It is critical to remember, however, that communication is the instrument by which physician and patient relate to each other and attempt to set and achieve therapeutic goals. In psychiatric care, the therapeutic agent is not the medication alone but the medication provided by the physician in the context of the physician-patient relationship. The quality and character of that relationship can significantly affect the outcomes of patient care and are essential to patients' satisfaction [9].

Elements of Effective Communication

At a very basic level, the physician needs first to hear the patient's 'story' [10]. Many physicians fear extended encounters when patients are allowed to talk, but focusing patients can help them to be succinct and clear. Failing to allow patients to tell their story curtails a valuable source of information about a patient; listening fully saves time in the long run [11]. The 'talking' therapies are obviously based on therapeutic communication, but the need for such therapeutic communication may not be obvious in medication-focused treatment. Considerable research suggests, however, that effective therapeutic communication involves listening to the patient's story well enough to offer treatment choices based not only on pharmacological action but also on what the patient believes and on what the patient can be expected to do [12].

Second, patients' responses to medical recommendations are also affected by the interpersonal aspects of their communication with their physicians, and in particular the trust that is built in the relationship [13]. Patients' reactions to psychiatric care in particular may be initially characterized by embarrassment and defensiveness. Empathic understanding of patients can ultimately lead to important health benefits [14, 15]. Emotional support of patients through long-term care as well as the encouragement of their healthier lifestyles depend upon apprehension of their emotions and responsiveness to their affective experiences. Physician empathy is essential to understand the utility of any proposed regimen to the patient, and the relationship of benefits to costs in the patient's estimation [16]. Rapport and the communication of emotional support through nonverbal communication skills can help to cement the physician's relationship with the patient, and their absence can hinder effective care [17].

Third, clarity of communication is essential for patients to understand the regimens to which they hope to adhere. Treatment information tends to be communicated to patients in a foreign code that may be difficult to understand [18]. Physicians in all specialties regularly use medical terms that patients do not understand, and patients are often too ill at ease and lack sufficient skills to articulate their questions [19]. Close to 50% of patients leave their doctors' offices not knowing what they are supposed to do to take care of themselves [17]. Further, when patients are doubtful about the utility of a medication, they may purposely ignore it or conveniently forget to take it.

Fourth, effective communication is essential to understanding the patient's evaluations of the value and efficacy of the recommendation, as well as the patient's expected (or experienced) practical limitations in carrying it out. Differences in physicians' and patients' expectations can significantly contribute to noncompliance or even the risk of malpractice litigation [12]. Effective communication allows the assurance of truly informed consent, with clear discussion of alternative therapies, expected benefits, risks, and direct and indirect costs.

What Patients Want from Their Physicians

The physician-patient relationship, in all specialties including psychiatry, has traditionally been based on physician dominance in the decisionmaking process. Influenced by the consumer movement, this relationship is gradually evolving into one of shared decisionmaking in which physicians and patients view themselves as collaborators [20]. Traditionally, defining the problem, setting health goals, and choosing among alternatives was done only by the physician, who then assigned the patient a treatment plan. More recently, however, patients have become more vocal in expressing their desire for personal control and choice in maximizing their health outcomes [21]. Many patients want to play an active role in their care, and need to trust the competence and truthfulness of their caregivers. Patients want respect for their values, preferences, and expressed needs, they want communication and education, coordination of their care, and attention to their physical comfort and quality of life. Patients also want emotional support and reassurance toward the alleviation of their fears and anxieties, involvement of their family where appropriate, and continuity of care or orderly and effective transition to another health professional [22, 23].

The most effective relationships between physicians and patients are those in which physician and patient share power and control of health care decisions

[24]. In practice, this sharing of power requires open, honest, and forthright conversation between physician and patient, sometimes toward the goal of resolving their conflicting goals and preferences. Without this communication, a genuinely collaborative relationship with the physician will be impossible, and without understanding how to resolve their inevitable minor conflicts, physician and patient will enter into a tacit collusion that conflict in their views does not, and cannot, exist.

Informed Consent and Informed Choice

Informed consent is an ethical and a legal concept that is central to the physician-patient relationship. It requires that the physician disclose to the patient in a truthful and nonmanipulative way information pertinent to an anticipated medical course of action. It also requires that the patient comprehend the information well enough to be able to make a voluntary choice that is free from force, coercion, or duress. 'Informed choice' takes this concept a step further, and requires that the patient is regularly provided with sufficient information about every relevant aspect of the medical condition and the options available for dealing with it. In light of the information they receive, patients are able to make informed choices about many steps in the process of their care [25].

Taking this concept a step further, it is suggested that informed collaborative choice (ICC) better suits today's patients than a traditional paternalistic model might, and one that fosters greater satisfaction and adherence [26]. ICC is based upon a relationship of mutual participation by physician and patient [27]. Together, physician and patient define the nature of the problem and together they determine and voice their expected outcomes. For the physician, this might be reducing the patient's depression; for the patient, it might be doing so without uncomfortable side effects. Patient and physician then engage in whatever task-oriented and socioemotional behaviors are necessary to communicate about these goal outcomes, each making sure his or her views are fully understood by the other. Physician and patient then communicate about the potential effect of various alternatives for dealing with the problem and achieving the stated outcome goals. Through the process of negotiation, they jointly decide on one of the alternatives (e.g. one or another prescription, behavioral modification, psychotherapy, or some combination of these) which, with a likelihood acceptable to the patient and physician, has a chance of accomplishing the decided-upon goals. Such an approach is consistent with models proposed in the literature such as negotiated patienthood [28], patient involvement [29] and patient participation [30].

ICC does not involve patients telling their physicians what to do; patients are highly unlikely to have physician domination as their goal [12]. Rather, while collaboration certainly involves the patient asserting the right to self-determination, it also involves compromise on the part of both parties: the patient does not engage in self-care alone, rejecting medical treatment, but rather works with the physician to try to achieve the agreed-upon health outcome goals.

Barriers to Physician-Patient Collaboration

Societal expectations and medical tradition, however, make it particularly difficult for patients to assert their needs for information, explanation, and collaboration. Patients want far more information than their physicians think they do, and far more detailed disclosures than their physicians usually offer to them [9, 31]. Further, physicians and patients tend to have widely different beliefs about what constitutes adequate disclosure: patients want extensive disclosures of risks and alternatives, whereas physicians generally provide very little information about these [31, 32]. Because of traditional concepts of the doctor-patient relationship, many patients respond to physician control with acquiescence; instead of asserting their needs to have their questions answered, patients may ignore their own concerns and state they will embark on regimens that they really have no intention of following or do not understand well enough to follow correctly. In clinical practice, physicians often assume that they know what their patients' preferences are, but they are mostly incorrect [21, 33]. In response to time and other practice pressures, physicians tend to make assumptions about patient preferences and make decisions for, instead of with, their patients.

Value of Conflict

When patients have equal decisionmaking power with their physicians, the possibility is opened up that the two will disagree with one another. In order to avoid this possibility, physicians are often tempted to present themselves as certain of the one right course, failing to divulge the range of options available for treatment and the uncertainty of each [34]. Further, a pattern of avoiding conflict may interfere with the exploration of adherence problems and foster ignorance of noncompliance as the reason for poor outcomes. A productive physician-patient relationship, on the other hand, requires the ability to work together to acknowledge the inevitability and the value of conflict and to work toward its resolution [35].

Benefits of ICC

ICC does not come naturally to physicians or to patients. It requires awareness and behavioral change, including effective communication, a conscious approach to the therapeutic relationship as collaboration, and a recognition of the patient's right to choose his or her own course of action [36]. Elements of communication in the context of ICC are associated with more adequate histories given by patients, with less delay in the timely reporting of important symptoms, and with greater overall patient satisfaction with care [37]. Collaboration and opportunities for informed choice also improve patients' sense of personal control over their health [38]. When physicians offer more information, and talk more with their patients about issues of adherence, their patients are more likely to adhere [39, 40]. Physicians' interpersonal manner can have important effects on patients' subsequent health behaviors as well as their acceptance or rejection of medical advice and appointment keeping [41].

Conclusion

The chronic nature of psychiatric conditions, and constraints on treatment time and health care resources require that patients become partners with their physicians in decisionmaking about their psychiatric care. Loss of decisionmaking power is a function of problems in communication in the physician-patient relationship. When patients try to regain that power through noncompliance, they waste costly medical care resources and may even jeopardize their health [42].

A physician-patient relationship without collaboration, negotiation, and the resolution of conflict falls short of an effective interchange. Physicians need to take the initiative to reassure their patients that disagreement between them may arise, and when it does they will work out their differences together [33]. Patient and physician need to view disagreement not as a threat or failure, but as a sign of active collaboration focused on the important goal of the patient's health and well-being.

References

1   Baldessarini RJ: Enhancing treatment with psychotropic medicines. Bull Menninger Clin 1994;58: 224–241.
2   Ruscher SM, de Wit R, Mazmanian D: Psychiatric patients' attitudes about medication and factors affecting noncompliance. Psychiatr Serv 1997;48:82–85.

3   Epstein LH, Cluss PA: A behavioral medicine perspective on adherence to long-term medical regimens. J Consult Clin Psychol 1982;50:950–971.

4   Boyd JR, Covington TR, Stanaszek WF, Coussons RT: Drug defaulting. I. Determinants of compliance. Am J Hosp Pharm 1974;31:362–366.

5   DiMatteo MR, DiNicola DD: Achieving Patient Compliance: The Psychology of the Medical Practitioner's Role. Elmsford, Pergamon, 1982.

6   Epstein LH: The direct effects of compliance on health outcome. Health Psychol 1984;3:385–393.

7   DiMatteo MR, Hays RD, Gritz ER, Bastani R, Crane L, Elashoff R, Ganz P, Heber D, McCarthy W, Marcus A: Patient adherence to cancer control regimens: Scale development and initial validation. Psych Assessment 1993;5:102–112.

8   Cassell EJ: The Theory of Doctor-Patient Communication. Cambridge, MIT, 1985.

9   Waitzkin H: Information giving in medical care. J Health Soc Behav 1985;26:81–101.

10   Kleinman A: The Illness Narratives: Suffering, Healing and the Human Condition. New York, Basic Books, 1988.

11   Beckman HB, Frankel RM, Darnley J: Soliciting the patient's complete agenda: A relationship to the distribution of concerns. Clin Res 1985;33:714A.

12   Roter DL, Hall JA: Doctors Talking with Patients/Patients Talking with Doctors: Improving Communication in Medical Visits. Westport, Auburn House, 1992.

13   Squier RW: A model of empathic understanding and adherence to treatment regimens in practitioner-patient relationships. Soc Sci Med 1990;30:325–339.

14   LeVasseur J, Vance D: Doctors, nurses, and empathy; in Spiro HM, Curnen MGM, Peschel E, St James D (eds): Empathy and the Practice of Medicine: Beyond Pills and the Scalpel. New Haven, Yale, 1993, pp 76–84.

15   Warner MS: Does empathy cure? A theoretical consideration of empathy, processing, and personal narrative; in Bohart AC, Greenberg LS (eds): Empathy Reconsidered: New Directions in Psychotherapy. Washington, American Psychological Association, 1997, pp 125–140.

16   Kleinman A, Eisenberg L, Good B: Culture, illness and care: Clinical lessons from anthropologic and cross-cultural research. Ann Intern Med 1978;88:251–258.

17   DiMatteo MR: The Psychology of Health, Illness and Medical Care: An Individual Perspective. Pacific Grove, Brooks/Cole,1991.

18   Christy NP: English is our second language. N Engl J Med 1979;300:979–981.

19   Roter DL: Patient question asking in physician-patient interaction. Health Psychol 1984;3:395–409.

20   Haug MR, Lavin B: Consumerism in Medicine: Challenging Physician Authority. Beverly Hills, Sage, 1983.

21   Kaplan RM: Health-related quality of life in patient decision making. J Soc Issues 1991;47:69–90.

22   Delbanco TL: Enriching the doctor-patient relationship by inviting the patient's perspective. Ann Intern Med 1992;116:414–418.

23   McBride CA, Shugars DA, DiMatteo MR, Lepper HS, O'Neil EH, Damush TM: The physician's role: Views of the public and the profession on seven aspects of patient care. Arch Fam Med 1994; 3:948–953.

24   Ballard-Reisch DS: A model of participative decision making for physician-patient interaction. Health Commun 1990;2:91–104.

25   Spaeth GL: Informed choice, not informed consent. Ophthalmic Surg 1992;23:648–649.

26   DiMatteo MR, Gambone JC, Reiter RC: Enhancing medication adherence through commun and collaborative informed choice. Health Commun 1994;6:253–265.

27   Szasz PS, Hollender MH: A contribution to the philosophy of medicine: The basic model of the doctor-patient relationship. Arch Intern Med 1956;97:585–592.

28   Lazare A, Eisenthal S, Frank A, Stoeckle J: Studies on a negotiated approach to patienthood; in Gallagher E (ed): The Doctor-Patient Relationship in the Changing Health Scene. Washington, USDHEW, 1978, pp 78–83,119–140.

29   Greenfield S, Kaplan S, Ware JE Jr: Expanding patient involvement in care: Effects on patient outcomes. Ann Intern Med 1985;102:520–528.

30   Speedling EJ, Rose DN: Building an effective doctor-patient relationship: From patient satisfaction to patient participation. Soc Sci Med 1985;21:115–120.

31 Faden RR, Becker C, Lewis C, Freeman J, Faden AI: Disclosure of information to patients in medical care. Med Care 1981;19:718–733.

32 Brody DS: The patient's role in clinical decision-making. Ann Intern Med 1980;93:718–722.

33 Katz J: The Silent World of Doctor and Patient. New York, Free Press, 1984.

34 Wolf, SM: Conflict between doctor and patient. Law Med Health Care 1988;16:197–203.

35 Freidson E: Professional Dominance. Chicago, Aldine, 1970.

36 Inui TS, Yourtee EL, Williamson JW: Improved outcomes in hypertension after physician tutorials: A controlled trial. Ann Intern Med 1976;84:646–651.

37 DiMatteo MR, Taranta A, Friedman HS, Prince LM: Predicting patient satisfaction from physicians' nonverbal communication skills. Med Care 1980;18:376–387.

38 Brody DS, Miller SM, Lerman CE, Smith DG, Caputo GC: Patient perception of involvement in medical care: Relationship to illness attitudes and outcomes. J Gen Intern Med 1989;4:506–511.

39 Eisenthal S, Emery R, Lazare A, Udin H: Adherence and the negotiated approach to patienthood. Arch Gen Psychiatry 1979;36:393–398.

40 Schulman BA: Active patient orientation and outcomes in hypertensive treatment: Application of a socio-organizational perspective. Med Care 1979;17:267–280.

41 DiMatteo MR, Hays RD, Prince LM: Relationship of physicians' nonverbal communication skills to patient satisfaction, appointment noncompliance, and physician workload. Health Psychol 1986; 5:581–594.

42 Hayes-Bautista DE: Modifying the treatment: Patient compliance, patient control and medical care. Soc Sci Med 1976;10:233–238.

M. Robin DiMatteo, PhD, Department of Psychology, University of California, Riverside, Riverside, CA–92521 (USA)
Tel. +1 909 787 5734, Fax +1 909 787 3985

Guimón J, Fischer W, Sartorius N (eds): The Image of Madness. The Public Facing Mental
Illness and Psychiatric Treatment. Basel, Karger, 1999, pp 231–238

....

Rethinking the Problem of Noncompliance in Chronic Mental Illness

Sally E. Thorne

School of Nursing, University of British Columbia, Vancouver, Canada

According to accepted wisdom within professional and scholarly mental health circles, noncompliance with medical recommendations has been understood as an irrational and even pathological behavioral response. Controlling access to services, patient education, and a range of supportive strategies are typically evoked to counteract noncompliance on the assumption that compliance will be associated with better outcomes and noncompliance, inevitably, with worse [1]. In this discussion, I intend to challenge that assumption. I will argue that the beliefs underlying the position of western biomedicine with regard to management of a range of chronic health challenges are ideological and problematic. On that basis, I will propose an interpretive but grounded construction of noncompliance that offers the possibility of new approaches to both clinical management and health care policy. Drawing upon recent shifts in our understanding of noncompliance derived from insider perspectives on what it is like to have a chronic physical disease, I will argue that the phenomenon referred to by professionals (and often by patients themselves) as 'noncompliance' can alternatively be understood as a strategic device in the lengthy and complex process of reworking a life narrative to accommodate disease, illness, and treatment implications into the business of living well.

In the domain of mental health practice and research, noncompliance with medical prescription has been addressed as a significant barrier to optimal treatment outcomes. Similarly, those working in the field of chronic physical illness have identified noncompliance in its own right as among the most serious and costly of modern health care problems [2]. The proliferation of research into the factors associated with noncompliance and the health beliefs with which it can be correlated reveals an enduring intensity about and fascination for the 'problem' that noncompliance represents [3, 4].

Interpretations of the Science

The clinical trials upon which all scientific 'proof' of a chemotherapeutic agent's efficacy are founded assume total compliance. However, insider research into a range of chronic illnesses reveals that full compliance with medical prescription is extremely rare indeed, even during clinical trials [5, 6]. Because subjects in studies of chemotherapeutic agents intended for long-term use and self-care management are rarely studied in controlled environments, such as would be the case for subjects of studies directed toward more acute health conditions, the noncompliance that is apparent in general chronic illness management is undoubtedly a major factor in clinical trials. Just as patients are unlikely to report noncompliance to professionals who would be displeased that their orders have been disregarded, noncompliance in clinical trials tends to remain invisible. It could be said, therefore, that what we actually know from our scientific study of effective drug management is based upon cardinal assumptions that cannot effectively be tested. However, paradoxically, we commonly conclude that absolute compliance with proven and standardized regimens is the only rational response for those who must self-manage a chronic disease condition.

Because we base our clinical strategies on such flawed assumptions about the science, the problem of noncompliance is almost universally understood as an intellectual, rational, social, or even moral failure within the individual patient [7–9]. Our clinical responses therefore include extensive support for intellectual knowledge acquisition (psychoeducation) and social reengineering (behavior modification, regimentation) to assist the individual toward overcoming such barriers and achieving the ideal of compliance. While practitioners in the field of chronic mental illness care may rationalize these approaches as an inherent product of primary disease manifestations (illogical thinking, delusions, forgetfulness, social irresponsibility and so on), they tend not to recognize that the same sorts of professional reasoning processes explain clinical approaches to physical diseases in which rational thought is unaltered by the effects of disease. Temporarily locating ourselves outside of these traditional assumptions about why we do what we do in mental illness care, it can be instructive to consider the meaning of noncompliance in physical illness as a model from which to deconstruct dominant western biomedical interpretations that may confound our ability to understand and respond to the way persons with chronic mental illness make sense of and order their lives.

Parallels in Chronic Physical Illness Ideology

I will illustrate this point by drawing upon findings from recent studies of patient decisionmaking in the context of a common physical illness, diabetes mellitus. Studies with individuals who have become expert in self-managing type 1 diabetes reveal that uncritical and compliant approaches to standardized insulin regimens turn out to be inconsistent with the highly attuned and reasoned approach that is required to live as well as possible over as long as possible a period with this complex disease [10, 11]. Our most recent research [Paterson and Thorne, unpubl. data] has involved qualitative investigation of the decisionmaking processes of 20 individuals determined by their medical specialists to be experts in self-management decisionmaking. Recognizing the seasonal nature of many of the decisions involved, each individual is being interviewed intensively several times over the course of a year. Further, a 'think-aloud' strategy has been employed, permitting participants to record the intricacies of their daily decisionmaking into a tape recorder for an entire week several times over the course of the year. Transcriptions from the think-aloud process are then used as a basis for increasing depth in subsequent interviews. Preliminary analysis of the data from this exhaustive study confirms that these patients report extensive manipulation of diet, exercise and insulin according to intensely complex and changing variables in both physiological response and life circumstance [12].

According to individuals who have developed this kind of expertise in self-management of diabetes, considerable experimentation and testing for variation are prerequisite to the achievement of excellence in complex decisionmaking. They must learn to notice subtle variations in sensation or response, to interpret and manage an extensive range of bodily cues, and to predict the implications that might derive from any one of a wide range of possible responses. This sophisticated and highly individualized knowledge upon which to base decisionmaking is gleaned not from compliance with treatment orders but rather from an extended and strategic pattern of what could well be termed 'experimental non-compliance'. The developmental trajectory toward expertise in self-management decisionmaking typically involves a range of actions and decisions that include such departures as 'cheating' on diets, risk taking with regard to serum glucose levels, and taking 'holidays' from the brutal routine of responsible daily self-management. While such departures represent defiance of medical orders and the very real threat of serious repercussions, they also provide a basis upon which an understanding of the complexities of interaction and effect can gradually be developed, modified, and reevaluated. As patients describe these processes, they reveal a thoughtful understanding of what biomedical science has to offer in support of their challenge combined with an acute awareness of its limitations. Whether they reveal such insights to the health professionals involved in their care depends largely on the degree to which they anticipate negative judgements about their strategies. Professionals capable of receiving information about such noncompliance without assuming it requires 'intervention' are reported to be rare indeed [6].

In keeping with the emerging knowledge from other studies in this field, these preliminary findings suggest that there are distinct patterns within this learning process, including periods in which departures from medical orders are more frequent and dramatic as well as other occasions during which more compliant patterns (at times even permitting professionals to control decisionmaking completely) may be strategic [12]. To date, the research demonstrates quite clearly that such learning is highly individualized to unique circumstances and physiologies. It seems probable that the intricate process of developing expertise in diabetes self-management decisionmaking takes a decade or more beyond diagnosis and initial treatment. In contrast, however, diabetes education programs worldwide typically strive to foster compliance with prescribed regimens and actively discourage experimentation with prescription and individualized adaptive learning. Toward this end, they often convey the message that noncompliance will inevitably lead to dire consequences in disease progression and complications [10], setting up conditions under which the patient's learning experiences place him or her in direct opposition to the efforts of the formal support systems. As the diabetes example prototypically illustrates, professional responses to the problem of outcomes in the management of many chronic physical illnesses have been largely based upon the prevailing philosophy of ensuring compliance with professional expert decisions rather than developing expert self-care decisionmaking skills within the patient [6]. Recognizing the degree to which such ideological orientations have influenced clinical practice and even health policy in the realm of physical illness care challenges the psychiatric community with documenting similar patterns in the context of chronic mental illness care.

The Problem of Complex Self-Care Management

Beyond the unmistakable distinction that persons with diabetes would normally be considered rational while persons with chronic schizophrenia would not, there are obvious parallels in the medical management of many chronic physical and mental illnesses. Both may involve powerful and potentially dangerous chemotherapeutic agents whose side effects can seriously impair quality of life. Both invoke physical and emotional symptomatology that can be extraordinarily subtle and difficult to interpret. And both involve a delicate balance between controlling the effects of the disease and controlling the effects of the treatment.

In the context of chronic illness of either a physical or a mental nature, the relevant outcome of the disease management process is a valued quality of life, a factor that is by definition highly subject to individual interpretation. Thus, when we think about how we know about the effects of compliance with treatment and how we measure the outcomes that we measure, clear difficulties emerge within the science. For example, while an isolative, rigidly controlled lifestyle might be ideal for one individual, the ability to be flexible, to interact socially, and to take risks might be indispensable to another. For the person with diabetes or schizophrenia alike, the professional health care system cannot simply assume an understanding of what a valued quality of life entails and therefore predetermine what compromises must be made in the process of achieving it.

When asked, individuals with chronic illnesses of all types typically report a wide range of noncompliant behaviors [6]. Where chemotherapy is involved, such noncompliance ranges from altered timing and dosage to periodic or even complete withdrawal from prescribed medications. The clinical and scientific response to the 'problem' of noncompliance consistently reveals three important assumptions: (1) that compliance is preferable to noncompliance, (2) that noncompliance is irrational, and (3) that controlling the factors consistent with noncompliance will correct the problem [5]. Since each assumption is of questionable validity, it seems that there are considerable grounds on which to challenge all of what we know and think about noncompliance and begin afresh. Thus, the argument is made that we ought to revisit the methods we use in our randomized controlled trials in an attempt to learn what patients actually do rather than simply recording what they say they do. Instead of assuming that noncompliance is inherently problematic, we should investigate its potential contributions to the learning trajectory within chronic illness management. And rather than accepting that our successful patients have been compliant where our less successful ones have not, I believe that we ought to reconsider the judgments inherent in our clinical conclusions and inquire more deeply into what it is that our successful patients learn that enables them to reconcile the adverse effects of psychotherapeutic agents with the complexities inherent in a life well lived.

Alternative Therapeutic Strategies

From a perspective of understanding noncompliance as a rational and strategic component of the complex learning involved in living well with a chronic illness, the clinician can begin to discern the possibility of new and liberating ways of interacting with patients. In contrast to the paternalism associated with viewing the professional as authority and the patient as reprobate, the clinical challenge in a chronic context becomes one in which the enthusiasm and expertise of each party are indispensable to the eventual health outcome. Instead of placing the emphasis on compliance, a more realistic approach involves recognizing the issue as one of balancing control of primary symptoms with the noxious side effects of chemical therapeutics. Instead of presuming that the problem confronting the patient is straightforward and logical, the professional who looks beyond traditional assumptions will understand the learning curve as extended and the challenge of developing expert decisionmaking skills as complex. Finally, rather than assuming that one can predict the best interests of clients, the creative practitioner will recognize that the only meaningful outcome measure in any clinical situation will be a valued quality of life – a quality of life that best represents the dreams, hopes and aspirations of that unique individual.

The trajectory of learning to manage a chronic mental illness with supportive chemotherapeutic measures will inevitably be long and difficult. If we approach supportive care from the perspective of a living model rather than a scientific model, we begin to understand that our primary obligation is to recognize the complexity of the challenge and to create processes that support and celebrate each hurdle our patients cross in meeting it. In contrast to the power struggles inherent in relationships that are based upon compliance, effective therapeutic alliances with our patients must be appreciated as fundamental to our capacity to assist *them* with *their* illness management. When health care professionals understand that patients are the expert in their own lives, and recognize that technical expertise related to the intervention is but one minor component within the complex puzzle of learning to live well with any chronic illness, then effective partnership emerges as the primary strategy for any therapeutic engagement.

Such therapeutic partnerships depend upon rethinking the meaning of compliance, and reframing the way we communicate about it to patients. If the clinician anticipates that the complex learning of bodily cues, emotional triggers, and unique response patterns will inevitably require experimentation, a relationship can be developed in which such experimentation is rendered visible and its processes and outcomes discussed openly. Such processes as manipulating medication dosage in order to be able to participate in valued activities or to experience valued feelings can become shared ideals rather than the secret acts of the patient alone. As the model of physical illness demonstrates, traditional communication strategies do not reduce noncompliance, they simply remove it from the clinician's line of vision. When clinicians take the lead and communicate an appreciation for the complexities of learning and the inherent individuality of each treatment plan, experimentation can become a negotiated process, and therefore more safe, productive, and effective. And as clinicians open up these avenues of communication, they will often find that their patients' decisions are based on accessible and respectable reasoning processes, even if they do on occasion contradict the prevailing unitary logic of biomedical science.

Conclusion

If we approach noncompliance as a rational component within a long and complex learning process whose ultimate endpoint can be envisioned by the patient alone, then our ability to engage with it nonjudgmentally, to interpret it within a broader context, and to support our patients as they learn to manage their illnesses will be greatly enhanced. Examination of the health professional and scientific ideologies embedded in the way we construct services for those with chronic physical illness provides us with an alternative perspective on how we might understand the decisions and actions we collectively refer to as 'noncompliance' among the chronically mentally ill. Thus, as we interrogate and deconstruct embedded assumptions such as those inherent in the noncompliance phenomenon, we create the means by which we might challenge traditional notions of social control of mental illness and replace them with mechanisms for understanding and supporting the everyday living processes of those members of our society who must face these particular challenges of the mind and body.

References

1   Dubyna J, Quinn C: The self-management of psychiatric medications: A pilot study. J Psychiatr Ment Health Nurs 1996;3:297–302.
2   Trostle JA: Medical compliance as an ideology. Soc Sci Med 1988;27:1299–1308.
3   Cameron C: Patient compliance: Recognition of factors involved and suggestions for promoting compliance with therapeutic regimens. J Adv Nurs 1996;24:244–250.
4   Wichowski HC, Kubsch SM: The relationship of self-perceptions of illness and compliance with health care regimens. J Adv Nurs 1997;25:548–553.
5   Thorne SE: Constructive noncompliance in chronic illness. Holistic Nurs Pract 1990;5:62–69.
6   Thorne SE: Negotiating Health Care: The Social Context of Chronic Illness. Thousand Oaks, Sage, 1993.
7   DiMatteo MR, DiNicola DD: Achieving Patient Compliance: The Psychology of the Medical Practitioner's Role. New York, Pergamon Press, 1982.
8   Farberow NL: Noncompliance as indirect self-destructive behavior; in Gerber KE, Nehemkis AM (eds): Compliance: The Dilemma of the Chronically Ill. New York, Springer, 1986.

9 Hingson RW: The physician's problems in identifying potentially non-compliant patients; in Barofsky I (ed): Medical Compliance: A Behavioral Management Approach. Thorofare, Slack, 1977.

10 Hernandez CA: The experience of living with insulin-dependent diabetes: Lessons for the diabetes educator. Diabetes Educ 1995;21:33–37.

11 Paterson BL, Sloan J: A phenomenological study of the decision-making experience of individuals with long-standing diabetes. Can J Diabetes Care 1994;18:10–19.

12 Paterson BL, Thorne S, Dewis M: Adapting to and managing diabetes. Image J Nurs Sch, in press.

Sally E. Thorne, RN, PhD, Professor, School of Nursing, University of British Columbia, Vancouver, BC V6T 2B5 (Canada)
Tel. +1 604 822 7482, Fax +1 604 822 7466

Author Index

Subject Index

Cooperative action, parent relationship with
  therapist 81
Cycle of disadvantage
  breaking 99–101
  points of intervention 99

Definition, initial recognition of mental
  illness 2, 3, 39
Depression
  causes, lay beliefs 24, 25
  comorbidity with other mental disorders
    119
  prevalence perception 27
  public knowledge in Switzerland 33
Drug addiction, public knowledge in
  Switzerland 34

Education
  effect on neighbors of facilities
    attitudes 108, 113, 114
    behavioral intentions 108, 109
    clinical implications 115
    confounding factors 113
    contact with staff and patients 109–111
    follow-up 108
    limitations 115
    patient illness, behavior, and social
      networks 111, 112
    patients' assessment 114
    recommendations 114, 115
    resistance to education campaign
      112, 113
    sociodemographic analysis of neighbors
      107
    study design 105–107
    supplementary questions 116
  impact on social acceptance 5, 6
  schizophrenia psychoeducational groups
    age differences 211–213
    assessment of patients 210
    compliance impact 213
    cost analysis 213, 214
    sex differences 210, 211
    study groups 209, 210
  stigma reduction programs 101–103
Employment, mentally ill
  estrangement 121, 122

programs 121, 122
Environment, cause of mental illness,
  perception 34, 35
Existential neurosis 119
Exposure
  effects on attitudes towards psychotropic
    drugs 176, 177, 183
  impact on social acceptance of mentally
    ill 6–8, 65, 130, 131

Family
  acceptance 4
  cause of mental illness, perception 34, 35
  neuroleptic attitudes 219, 220
  parental attitudes of child mental illness
    attitude towards professionals 74–77
    compatibility between lay and
      professional knowledge 77–80, 83
    questioning therapeutic relationship
      80–82
    study design 73
  significance of perceptions 1
  support groups 138, 140–142
Family crisis homes, domestic alternatives to
  hospitals 124
Functional logic 78

GRAAP support group
  attitudes towards neuroleptics
    doctor-patient relationship 217–219
    family member attitudes 219, 220
    side effects and offsetting benefits 217
    weight of experience 216, 217
  creation 138
  goals 140–142
  importance of self-help groups 221
  staff 142
Group therapy
  drug compliance improvement of patients
    149, 150
  efficacy 129
  medical students, attitude modification
    towards mentally ill
    authoritarianism 132–135
    overview of changes 132
    rationale 130, 131
    study design 131, 132, 135

schizophrenia psychoeducational groups
    age differences 211–213
    assessment of patients 210
    compliance impact 213
    cost analysis 213, 214
    sex differences 210, 211
    study groups 209, 210
    sensitization groups 129

Health professionals, *see also* Medical
    students
    acceptance 4, 5
    exposure impact on acceptance 6, 7, 57
    physician-patient relationship
        barriers to collaboration 227
        communication elements 224, 225
        GRAAP support group feedback
            217–219
        importance 223, 224
        informed collaborative choice 226–228
        informed consent 226
        patient needs 225, 226
        therapeutic partnerships 235–237
        value of conflict 227
    public underestimation of need 29
    significance of perceptions 1
The Heights, cooperative housing program
    126

Identification, initial recognition of mental
    illness 2, 3, 39
Informed collaborative choice
    benefits 228
    overview 226, 227
Informed consent 226
Institutional neurosis 119
Intervention, mental illness
    community intervention in treatment 3
    public attitudes and intervention
        preferences
        coherence of representations 50, 51
        deviant situations 54
        differentiation in forms according to
            situation 41, 42, 50
        favored forms 42, 43
        lay counsellors 43–45
        physician 45–47, 53

psychiatrist 45, 47–49, 52, 53
questionnaire design 40
social connotations 51, 52

Letting go logic 82

Madness
    images evoked 139
    meaning of term 138, 139
    stigma 139, 140
Mania, lay definition 62, 64, 66
Meaninglessness, feelings of mentally ill
    118, 119
Medical students
    attitude modification towards mentally ill
        with group therapy
        authoritarianism 132–135
        overview of changes 132
        rationale 130, 131
        study design 131, 132, 135
    mental illness attitudes 64
    psychotropic drug attitudes
        changes during undergraduate medical
            education 189–192, 194, 195
        open question responses 188, 189
        perception of attitude questions
            193, 194
        rationale for study 187
        relevance in compliance 188
        side effects 191, 192, 195
    schizophrenia word associations
        21, 22
Medication, *see* Psychotropic drugs
Metaphor, illness
    AIDS 13, 14, 19
    cancer 13, 14, 19
    schizophrenia
        mystification 17, 18
        overview 13–17, 19
        terror of the word 14, 15
    tuberculosis 13, 14, 17, 19

Normlessness, feelings of mentally ill
    121

Paranoid schizophrenia, *see* Schizophrenia
Parent, *see* Family
